Worshipping Your Wife 2

Best of the Blog

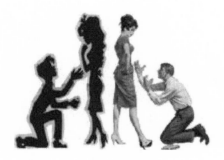

Mark Remond

Lulu.com

Also by Mark Remond:
*Worshipping Your Wife: Six Steps for Turning Marriage
Back Into Passionate Courtship* (Lulu, 2008)

ISBN 978-0-557-40725-5

Printed in the United States of America

This book is a selection of my posts and readers' comments to
my blog, "Worshipping Your Wife," from 2007 to early 2010.
Posts are arranged by topic rather than chronological sequence.
Due to space constraints, I have been able to include only a tiny
sampling of comments (and not necessarily those I agree with);
these were all posted anonymously or pseudonymously, and
many have been further disguised and edited for space and,
occasionally, content.

I welcome questions and comments on my blog,
http://worshippingyourwife.blogspot.com, or by email:
markremond@yahoo.com

For my wife
and my readers

*"When the wife is in charge,
things go well and love is in the air."*

—Unknown

Table of Contents

ACKNOWLEDGMENT:
A TRIBUTE TO LADY 'M'

(4.17.08)

In my book I celebrate the rise of FLRs, female-led relationships, and LFA, loving female authority:

"…a new type of female empowerment—not to be confused with female domination or female supremacy. In fact, the proponents of this new empowerment generally dismiss the world of 'femdom,' with its bizarre rituals and iconography, as a kind of male-oriented fantasyland, in which women are ultimately devalued." (*Worshipping Your Wife*, p. 84)

I don't know who coined the terms FLR and LFA, but the acronyms have definitely taken hold, especially FLR, helping to destigmatize and advance the cause of women as loving leaders in marriages and romantic relationships.

They've accomplished this largely by replacing all the mondo bizarro imagery associated with "femdom"—B&D, S&M, *et al.* Instead of a whip-wielding, vinyl-sheathed dominatrix lording it over a groveling lump of naked male flesh, we may now envision something akin to the radiant image that graces Lady

1

Misato's website, "Real Women Don't Do Housework"—and also the cover of my book.

"The Accolade" (1901) by Edmund Leighton depicts a lovely queen or princess, standing statuesque in a shaft of light as she confers knighthood with a longsword on a kneeling, unhelmeted warrior, head bent. Googling will yield many similar images from Leighton, along with those by his fellow historical painters in the English Pre-Raphaelite school, John William Waterhouse and Sir Edward Burne-Jones.

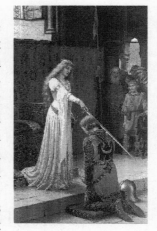

Yes, submissive men can be viewed as heroic knights, and their dominant damsels may be transfigured as radiant and fully empowered queens. This is not just the storybook romance model, but the courtship model, which Lady Misato converted into a working blueprint for contemporary wife-worship (or "wifedom," as she also calls it) and which I subsequently made the cornerstone of my book.

I acknowledge my considerable debt to Fumika Misato, not just for inspiring my book, but also for helping to save my marriage—and many other marriages, I'm sure. Perhaps she did not originate the terms "Loving Female Authority" (that may have been Elise Sutton, softening her own website a bit) and "Female Led Relationship," but "Wife Worship" is almost certainly Lady Misato's inspired coinage. And I regard her as the prime creatrix of the new FLR movement, which is rapidly gaining mainstream acceptance.

For me, and many other men I have discussed these matters with, it was "Real Women Don't Do Housework" that showed us that our longings to serve a woman are neither twisted nor perverse, but are at the very pulsing heart of romantic longing, even of heroic courtship. They can be proclaimed proudly, not hidden away or denied. Instead of leading us into masturbatory fantasies over kinky images, these longings can lead us right back into our marriages and back to our wonderful wives. We have only to embrace our wives as loving leaders, to treat them as the queens and goddesses they truly are.

Or, to cite my favorite motto: "If you want your wife to be a goddess, worship her."—Clairette de Longvilliers

INTRODUCTION:
A SHORT COURSE IN WIFE WORSHIP

For those who have not read my book, here is a 750-word Cliff Notes-type version:

WORSHIPPING YOUR WIFE: Six Steps for Turning Marriage Back Into Passionate Courtship

"Boyfriends need to understand that if women are worshipped, the world will be a better place." —Nicole Kidman

"The thrill is gone."

It's the lament of so many married couples. Husbands and wives drift apart, physically and emotionally, or maintain alliances of custom and convenience, keepers of a flickering flame.

Love has its seasons, as John Gray reminds us in *Men Are From Mars, Women Are From Venus*. It's folly to expect eternal springtime, perpetual romance.

But what if it's not necessarily true? What if love can be rekindled, even the all-consuming passion of first love? And not rekindled briefly, for just a season, but "ever after," creating that fairytale future couples dream about when saying their vows?

That's the extravagant claim of *Worshipping Your Wife: Six Steps for Turning Marriage Back Into Passionate Courtship*. Yes, courtship—because that's when guys and girls find each other most mysterious and magnetic.

Here's the entire six-step program in a nutshell—nominally addressed to husbands, but most effective when hand-delivered by their wives (or girlfriends), with salty or salient passages underlined.

The husband needs to:

Step 1: Realize that "the thrill is gone" and that he wants to get it back.

A man will do anything to win the woman of his dreams. Should he lose her, he will do anything to win her back. Why, then, is he not willing to do anything, on a daily basis, to keep her contented? Because husbands don't perceive that a wife can be lost if never again wooed or won, that marriage is also a crisis, deserving of extreme efforts.

Step 2: Save His Sex Energies for His Wife.

The dirty little secret is that passion doesn't ebb, magic doesn't vanish—not for most husbands anyway. Their fantasy life continues unabated, only focused away from their wives. With visual erotica a mouseclick away, too many husbands, while technically faithful, yield to imaginary infidelity. And, at the risk of sounding Victorian, chronic masturbation, solo and secretive, can rob a marriage of its binding energies.

Step 3: Make *Her* His Fantasy

The solution is for the husband to make his wife the centerfold of his inflamed imagination, as she was during courtship. When a husband begins treating her with that same homage, the deadening scales of familiarity will dissolve and he will see her restored to full, feminine mystery and radiance.

Step 4: Court Her Every Day, Attempt to Win Her Anew

Let the dragon-slaying, and sonnet-making, and gift-giving continue. Also: In courtship, the man proclaims his romantic ever-readiness, but the woman decides when (or if) sex will happen. It is a wonderfully workable formula, attuned to the dynamics of male and female sexuality. Let the man be hopeful all day long, striving to earn or seduce ultimate favors. Let the

5

wife initiate and announce the main event ("Gentlemen, start your engines!"). Sex will be better and hotter for both—and more frequent.

Step 5: Pamper Her and Pitch in Around the House

Is it unmanly to pamper your wife? Is it insulting, or infantilizing to open doors for her when she's perfectly capable herself? Should a husband stick to gender-specific chores—washing the car, hauling out the garbage? The courtship model makes quick work of such debates: You can't do enough for her! And, in today's two-income marriages, the woman ought not be expected to tie on the apron the minute she parks her briefcase. Let her log a few after-work hours in the La-Z-Boy (with a magazine and a Merlot). It may pay erotic dividends later that night.

Step 6: Dare to Be Known by Her

Most men aren't comfortable discussing intimate or emotional issues—even sexual fantasies. But the more a marriage returns to the courtship model, the more a husband's thoughts—and fantasies—turn to his wife during the day, the more he will have to share with her at night (or other private times). Opening up to her will serve to strengthen emotional and sexual bonding—and preclude any temptation for a "misunderstood" husband to unburden himself to another woman.

Summing Up

"To me it's pretty simple," began a memorable post I found in a wife-worshipping message board. "It's all about doing what I can do to make my wife happy. Because when *she's* happy, *I'm* happy. It doesn't take much once you get the hang of it. Every single day I just pretend we are dating and I try to win her heart."

1

COURTSHIP RESUMED

Marriage Is No Excuse (8.25.08)

When I was a boy, it seemed like all the famous TV standup comics (men-only in those days) relied on marriage jokes. These were endless variations on Henny Youngman's classic "Take my wife... please!" (Like: "I take my wife everywhere, but she keeps finding her way back.")

Henny, Milton Berle, Shecky Greene, Alan King, Rodney Dangerfield, even non-Catskill-trained Midwestern comics like George Gobel, they all treated marriage as a joke.

"Some people claim that marriage interferes with romance. There's no doubt about it. Anytime you have a romance, your wife is bound to interfere."—Groucho Marx

But they didn't invent this particular shtick. Odysseus probably made Penelope jokes to his cronies, after he drove off the suitors. And the '50s and '60s anti-monogamy monologists were tame compared to earlier satirical icons, like the widly misanthropic American Ambrose Bierce, or the naughtily philanthropic Oscar Wilde, to wit:

"Bigamy is having one husband or wife too many. Monogamy is the same." —Oscar Wilde

7

"One should always be in love. That is the reason one should never marry."—Oscar Wilde, *A Woman of No Importance*

"Love: a temporary insanity, curable by marriage."
—Ambrose Bierce, *Devil's Dictionary*

So the standup guys were hardly blazing any trails, even for their time. As the '50s gave way to the '60s and '70s, free love became a worldwide rallying cry for youth, breaking loose from all conventional constraints. It was echoed by shrieking rocker and whispery folksinger alike.

The conventional attitude about no-commitment "rolling stone" relationship was perfectly reflected in John Hartford's lyrics for "Gentle on My Mind," made famous by Glen Campbell:

> *...it's knowin' I'm not shackled*
> *By forgotten words and bonds*
> *And the ink stains that have dried upon some line*
> *That keeps you in the back roads*
> *By the rivers of my memory*
> *That keeps you ever gentle on my mind*

I never quite bought into this massively indoctrinated prevailing wisdom, whether expressed by Borscht Belters or shaggy-haired troubadours. In my private recesses, I always believed in the happy-ever-after marriage, all evidence to the contrary notwithstanding (especially including my own parents' dysfunctional union).

In fact, I continued to believe in this storybook ideal even when my own marriage began to fall, well, a wee bit short. It should work in real life. After all, it did work in the kind of stories I liked to read, and to write. At least up to that final fadeout.

But maybe I was wrong, and all the cynical voices were right. Maybe marriage *is* an unnatural state.

"Monogamy is like reading the same book over and over."—Mason Cooley

"Love at first sight is easy to understand; it's when two people have been looking at each other for a lifetime that it becomes a miracle."—Amy Bloom

It was the revolutionary concept of the "courtship marriage," as described by Fumika Misato on her "Real Women Don't Do Housework" website, that suddenly stripped the scales from my eyes. "This," she declared flatly, "is a marriage in which your husband courts you till death does you part."

Such a sweet revelation! The secret to happy-ever-aftering is simply to let the courtship continue! What a wonderful gift Lady Misato had given me (and all of us). Through her, I experienced a complete restoration of my naïve and boyish faith in storybook romance.

Later on, doing a bit of research into the origins of courtly love, I came across this quote from a 13th century writer, a quote that, for me, carried more truth than all the collected matrimonial wisdom of Marx (G.), Wilde, Bierce, Youngman, *et al.*:

"Marriage is no excuse for not loving."—Andreas Cappellanus: *The Art of Honorable Love*, 13th century

Morale: If you want to keep the romance in your marriage, let the pre-nupt be that the husband continues to press his suit post-nupt, dill death do you part.

My own embrace of Lady Misato's advice radically transformed my marriage for the better, starting with my own attitude, and then, gradually, working its ways and wiles upon my wife. Granted, she was a little taken aback at first to find herself being courted again, but she's gotten to like it.

That transformation prodded me into writing a book, which I launched first on a website, then in publication.

As I wrote in an early draft, "The extravagant claim of this book is that love can be rekindled, even the all-consuming passion of first love. Not by returning to the time-tested, give-and-take practices of successful marriages (as most counselors recommend), but by the husband going all the way back to the giddy, unbalanced behaviors of courtship."

Courtship is such an exhilarating state, it turns out, that husbands and wives alike are euphoric to be in it, over and over again.

It's called being in love.

Happily Shackled (1.7.09)

"...And it's knowin' I'm not shackled / By forgotten words and bonds / And the ink stains that have dried upon some line... / That keeps you ever gentle on my mind."—John Hartford, "Gentle on My Mind"

Of course, it's precisely the contractual shackling of the wandering, marauding male animal that makes civilization (and wife worship) possible. "It's the miracle of love—and commitment," as I wrote in Chapter One of my book, citing a favorite quote from author George Gilder's seminal work, *Men and Marriage*:

"Women manipulate male sexual desire in order to teach men the long-term cycles of female sexuality and biology on which civilization is based."

Yes, manipulate. Hence, the wife-led marriage. It's not just comic relief, watching Fred Flintstone getting his daily comeuppance from Wilma. Nor is this domestic role reversal, with the wife calling the shots, contrary to the natural order of things.

I don't think it's going too far to say that the "perpetual courtship" or wife-worship or wife-led marriage is really what marriage is intended to be—the daily undertaking by the husband to make good on all those high-flown, ultra-romantic promises he repeated before he got to kiss the bride.

For the wife-worship husband, every day is promise-keeping day, with "love," "honor" and "cherish" atop his perennial to-do list—and "obey," as well, for a growing number of worshipful husbands.

Looking through saved web postings on these intimate matters, I came across the following, attributed only to a "Ms. Justine":

"In order for a male to fully be a man he must come under the full influence and control of a woman. The contract of marriage guarantees what the male animal most deeply longs for—to empty his testes on a regular basis. In exchange for this simple favor, he must surrender all that he thinks and knows as freedom. No longer can he do as he pleases. He must now work hard and be productive. Men only become loyal, faithful and productive when they come under the control of a woman. It is only the contract of marriage which insists that a man work and surrender the fruits of his labor."

George Gilder, I doubt not, would agree.

But, in John Hartford's terms, can't a guy "just leave my sleepin' bag / Rolled up and stashed behind your couch"? Does he have to be matrimonially bonded and shackled?

I dealt with this at some length in the previous posting, "Marriage Is No Excuse," but the short answer is, "Pretty much, yep."

Fumika Misato, creator of the provocative "Real Women Don't Do Housework" website, explains that while it is certainly possible for a woman to be worshipped within a long-term non-marital arrangement, "outside of marriage, there is (a) a temptation on the part of the man to seek an easier resolution, and b) no committed relationship into which to invest."

He needs, in other words, to be shackled. Happily, even blissfully shackled, if you ask me.

Appreciating Your Life—and Your Wife (7.3.08)

"Look at me one minute as though you really saw me... Doesn't anyone ever realize life while they live it? Every, every minute?"—Emily Webb in Thornton Wilder's *Our Town*, Act 3

Try to recall the most intense desire you have ever had for the woman who is now your wife. Perhaps during courtship, or on your honeymoon or a romantic vacation interlude.

When this she-creature was absolutely everything to you. When you could see the whole rest of your life in her eyes.

Or how about the intensity of feelings if you ever thought you could lose her forever? Maybe this never happened, but if it did, you'll know what I'm talking about.

Panic. Fear. A willingness to do anything to get her back, to change her mind, to make things okay again, the way they were before you screwed up royally (which I think we can safely assume you did). To crawl over broken glass, if that would do it, bearing flowers. To promise anything, do anything.

Even to give up televised sports. (Well, maybe not *that* far.)

Got it? That's how you really feel about your wife. So why not live that way, every day—"every, every minute?"

Disagree? Perhaps you think your honeymoon or courtship phase was less real, sort of an embarrassing, make-believe interlude better left to scrapbooks, syrupy Hallmark cards and old wedding videos.

But you'd be wrong. Not being attuned to those core feelings is the illusion. Taking your wife for granted is the pretend phase, imagining that other endeavors outrank her and her needs on your daily priority list.

She is really and truly your No 1. In fact, she's your perennial Top 10—and more.

And you don't need to wait for a crisis to realize it.

"Courtship and reconciliation are clearly defined crises in a man's life. He will do anything to win the woman of his dreams; should he lose her, he will do anything to win her back. Why, then, is he not willing to do anything, on a daily basis, to keep her contented? Because husbands don't perceive that a wife can be lost if never again wooed or won, that marriage is also a crisis, deserving of extreme efforts."—From the Introduction to *Worshipping Your Wife*

But, of course, sometimes it does takes a crisis for a husband to suddenly realize what matters most in his life—namely, his wife.

Such moments can be true "conversion" experiences, when the scales fall off one's eyes and one is forever changed.

Like this husband's conversion:

"Once I realized my wife wanted to leave me, I knew I was powerless. There was no way I could make her stay. I knew the only way she would stay would be if she was happy, and so I resolved to do whatever it took to make her happy... Part of the process involved giving up control of the marriage... I discovered that making my focus my wife and her happiness not only made the marriage better for her, but also for me."

And this one:

"Our marriage had hit the deepest crisis in its history. I'm sure that if I had not found your site [Lady Misato's "Real Women Don't Do Housework"], my marriage would have been unretrievable. I realized that radical changes had to be made. I found myself about 3 a.m. looking at my wife asleep on the bed... and suddenly it dawned upon me what I had to do! I began kissing her feet passionately and found that I'd unconsciously totally surrendered and submitted my life to her in a split second of impulse. From that moment on I was her obedient, willing-to-please husband."

No matter how incandescent the moment, of course, split-second impulses mean little if real and sustained change does not ensue, like this:

"I now take breakfast up to her every morning in bed, I'm doing all the housework, all the chores, cooking for her every night, she now controls our finances, my sexual relief, and I'm loyally obeying her, I have never been this happy, not ever, and I mean not ever. Our marriage has taken a 180 degree turn. She is my reason for living now and I kneel at her feet."

So, yes, it *can* happen. Happy-ever-aftering *is* possible. A husband and wife can really live this way.

Or not.

Comments:

Enoch: You are right, the shock of possibly losing your wife is a real eye-opener. For me it was a moment of absolute clarity when everything stood in sharp relief. It was suddenly crystal-clear what was important and what wasn't. And it has led to a life that I could never have imagined, but is what I always wanted!

Mark: I also have had moments akin when I realized who, and what, really mattered most in my life. The trick is to hold fast to that truth, to wear it like a wedding ring.

Susan's Pet: I recall the time, as you put it, "Or how about the intensity of feelings if you ever thought you could lose her forever?" We were married only a few months. She had pains. I would have given my life to spare her the suffering. It turned out well at the end. Now, decades later, I feel the same. She is my life.

Wife-Worship Syndrome (5.27.08)

Okay, maybe wife worship *is* just a bit offbeat. Maybe husbands aren't supposed to get stuck in perpetual courtship mode. Some wives might say, "Enough already with the flowers and gold Godiva boxes, all the pedicures and footrubs. Take me for granted, please, why dontcha?"

Maybe.

But if so, as personality syndromes go, this one has got to be pretty darned benign. And, unless the affected hubby is really relentless in his ministrations, his wife is unlikely to complain about all the amorous attentions. More likely is she to complain if they're suddenly discontinued.

Suddenly she is seen plainly, wrinkles and all, and no longer transfigured as a goddess. What happened, she might wonder, to those rose-colored glasses he'd taken to wearing around the house? Is it a bad thing to be beautified by the eye of the beholder you're married to? Couldn't a wife get used to that kind of amorous impairment in her man?

In my book (chapter 5, page 38), I touch on this briefly: "My wife accused me of having a foot fetish," said one [husband], "but I told her no, I have a wife fetish."

"By their fruits ye shall know them. Do men gather grapes of thorns, or figs of thistles?" (*Matthew* 7:16)

With effects so pleasingly benign, the aberrant condition of wife worship may be infinitely preferable to the ho-hum-drummery of marital normalcy.

Comments:

Enoch: I frequent a vanilla marriage message board, and I recall a complaint from a woman from a couple of years ago that her husband was a workaholic. Her comment was "I wish he was a wifeaholic."

Mark: When I was first thinking of doing the book, I pitched the title and concept to a female writer friend. "Oh, fantastic, a book on uxoriousness! I wish my husband would read it!"

Enoch: I have a big vocabulary, but that's one I didn't know. I'll definitely remember it and maybe slip it into conversation with my wife!

Turkey vs. Groundhog (5.20.08)

Groundhog Day? Not the holiday I'd pick for endless repetition. I opt for Thanksgiving instead. And, no, not because I want to OD on turkey and tryptophan in perpetuam.

It's because the act of giving thanks, over and over, day after day, never palls. It renews. Thanksgiving is the most basic of prayers. Before petitioning the Almighty for any boon, you should first acknowledge your blessings.

End of sermonette.

Because this post is about wife worship, not moral obligation. And gratitude also happens to be the starting point for wife worship. The worshipful husband gives thanks, each and every day, for the miraculous presence in his life of the woman who is his wife.

Life without her is not unimaginable. He can imagine it all right, and it's a wasteland! But God, or the Goddess, has given her to him. Or, to juggle the grammar to make it come out right, the God or Goddess has given him to her. And that is another act that the husband can affirm each day, giving himself to his wife, again and again.

"Each morning I try to declare my dedication, homage and gratitude to my wife," a husband writes. "I look into her beautiful eyes and tell her I love her. Then I kneel and kiss her feet. After kissing her feet I remain on my knees and thank her for allowing me to be her husband, for making my life wonderful, for making me the luckiest man. It's always an expression of gratitude... and I always mean it."

Amen to that. I wish I could institute that particular ritual in my own domestic agenda. From time to time I've been able to do it. but not on a daily basis.

Another man lectures on the importance of husbands' showing their gratitude to their wives: "A drink, a snack, a kiss, a caress... These are all signs of gratitude... If she assigns you a task, do it immediately, to the best of your ability, and thank her for the opportunity to serve her."

"Be patient, be obedient, reverent, grateful and attentive," adds another. "When my wife lets me make love to her, I always do it with much gratitude. I am the luckiest man I know. There is nothing I could do in twenty lifetimes to deserve such a gift."

The grateful male chorus continues: "I will never take my wife for granted. I will be mindful of how lucky I am to have her and seek a thousand little ways to express my gratitude."

Here's a husband who realizes it is not an easy thing for a wife to assume the leadership responsibility in a marriage: "Be sure to express that happiness and gratitude for her leadership and dominance. Ask for her leadership but don't dump responsibilities on her if she is not ready. I make a point to thank my wife for taking certain responsibilities and providing leader-ship—'Thank you for taking leadership on finding daycare for our daughter.' I thank her for correcting me, too."

I conclude with three quotations from women, beginning with pioneering female supremacist Elise Sutton. "You are a truly blessed man," she advises a husband whose wife is quickly as-suming command of their marriage. "So count those blessings and show your gratitude by increasing your efforts in serving your superior wife in a manner that she can appreciate and en-joy."

Paige Harrison offers similar counsel to husbands, not only those in acknowledged FLRs, but all husbands:

"Males must recognize and acknowledge that they are fortu-nate to be with a Woman. Those males who are wed and married should express their gratitude frequently and thank the Woman in their lives frequently." In particular, Harrison says, "If her body has borne children, he should praise her for all she has given."

"If every husband showed this kind of devotion and gratitude to his wife," writes a contented and well-worshipped wife, "divorces would be very rare!"

Comments:
Enoch: I constantly tell my wife how grateful I am for her. I thank her not only for her role in our family and her presence in my life, but also for not leaving me when she had every reason in the world to do so. (Like the hus-band you quoted, I kiss her feet on all fours every evening, too!) I tell her every day that I'm the luckiest man in the world. At first, she told me she was lucky too, but nowadays she answers me, "Yes, you *are* the luckiest man in the world."

Stuck on Courtship (8.6.08)

In case you somehow missed the message... This blog, and the book it's based on, both trumpet a return to courtship. And not just a return, mind you, but a return from which there is no return.

"Perpetual Courtship" I call it in Chapter Three:

"Thick-headedness and primal hunting instinct may convince a man that once he has been accepted by a woman, the chase is over. But it isn't—as husbands often discover too late, only when wives announce they're leaving—weary, perhaps, not so much of being mistreated as being treated indifferently. Brides can be won, and brides can be lost—if not courted and captivated anew each day. The chase, in other words, needs to be perpetual, with a daily quota of thrills and tribulations."

But (to argue the point) isn't that turning marriage, which should be a progression of life phases (what Gail Sheehy famously called "Passages") into an endless replay of the same passage. like a needle stuck in a groove (for readers old enough to remember the Vinyl Era)? What's the point of endlessly repeating one phase, even a happy phase, like in Groundhog Day? Isn't this turning pursuit of the love object into a closed-loop Sisyphean task, like Wily Coyote's pursuit of Roadrunner, Elmer Fudd's after Porky, Tom's after Jerry?

Don't we all want to move on in life? And does everything in life have to be about the woman? Catering to her, treating every day like a first date with a fistful of roses? What about guy stuff?

The simple answer is that perpetual courtship is designed for guys, as much as gals (to use a proscribed word I happen to like). The male animal craves the courtship phase. That's where he is most fully engaged. Doesn't matter if he's already married, the hunting-pursuing need is still there.

Take that ritual away and he is going to start straying. He will find his courtship elsewhere, outside the marriage, seeking strange flesh.

So, if you want to save or safeguard a marriage, keep the husband's courtship compulsion endlessly focused on his wife.

But doesn't the perpetual chase, with the quarry seemingly always beyond his reach, make a husband frustrated or insecure? A wee bit, sure. But it also makes him more ardent. "On the edge," as Lady Misato puts it. Certainly it makes marriage, and life, more exciting.

In a romantic courtship marriage, the ardent knight is always entering the lists against a new challenger, or riding out to prove his mettle against a new dragon. Motivation is always there. His Lady Fair is always enthroned or empedestaled, endlessly to be won—or lost.

What better authority to cite on courtship than two Loving Female Authorities, Fumika Misato and Elise Sutton?

Lady Misato: "The key to rediscovering courtship in marriage is to withdraw the certainty of romance. This simple idea leads to all sorts of interesting and exciting directions."

Elise Sutton: "During the courtship, a man has to gain permission from the woman if he can touch her or kiss her. Men treat women with more respect during the courtship than during the marriage because men soon take the woman for granted. The dominant woman always keeps the upper hand by making intimacy a reward and not a husbandly right. After all, the female body is a masterpiece and only a man full of reverence should be entitled to touch his Goddess."

I Get Letters (11.21.08)

A blog reader named Steve asks, "One question that I have is that many women feel uncomfortable being put up on a pedestal. How does a man deal with this?"

Good question, Steve, and one I'm still wrestling with in my own wife-worship marriage. I tell you, it was a pretty awkward and non-sequitur moment when, after ten years of conventional marriage, I suddenly dragged that stubby, Corinthian-capped pedestal into the living room, placed a small utility ladder beside it and encouraged her to climb up and be worshipped as a domestic goddess.

My bride categorically rejected the notion of female superiority or female dominance. She is a very egalitarian person, and indeed is very proud of my accomplishments, such as they are. "Don't be a sycophant!" she scolded me once, when I apparently was getting a bit too servile, carried away with a campaign of what is often called "stealth submissiveness."

And we husbands, newly converted to the gospel of wife-worship, can go to extremes. As I wrote in my book (Chapter 5, "Pampering and Pitching In"), "Are we getting slightly carried away? Advocating a kind of chivalrous silliness—opening doors and standing when she enters a room? Traditional feminists routinely label such masculine behavior as infantilizing, even insulting."

So I dragged that pedestal back out to the garage with the old cobwebbed exercise equipment. And I've learned in the decade since to curb my courtly impulses, not to throw my cloak over every encroaching mud puddle. I walk a fine line these days when it comes to catering to, or anticipating her wishes.

The trick for me is to do her bidding in a kind of macho, easygoing way. Call it the Moving Van guy, nodding when the lady of the house tells him where to set down the dresser he's hefting and what to bring out of the van next and where to put it.

If she sees me calmly alter my course, from whatever I'm doing in order to comply with her request, without the usual husbandly delaying tactics, she'll eventually get the desired message—that she is controlling me. I am, in other words, her servant, and she certainly realizes now that she has only to express a wish and I comply. Just so long as I don't act in what she regards as an unmanly way.

And that, I think, is what Lady Misato's Queen-Knight metaphor is all about. Courtliness. Being milady's champion, not her lackey. Milady's knight in combat, her dragon-slayer in chief.

To quote a husband who put that paradigm into daily practice, "I believe this is why the Knight-Queen analogy is so popular. Although the knight is subordinate to his Queen, he is still expected to retain the traditional 'manly-man' role to her of providing strength, security, and protection."

And, yes, there is a pedestal inherent in that Knight-Queen or Knight-Lady dynamic. He kneels before her, which does result in an incremental elevation of her status. Again, the trick is to ratchet up that elevation just a millimeter at a time, till eventually she's up where she belongs, regally empedestaled.

Again to quote my book (Chapter 3, "Perpetual Courtship"), "What wife can hold out against continuous, insidious courtship? How can she not be susceptible?"

As the oft-quoted (by me) Au876 put it, "...most if not all women love to be pampered, adored, worshipped and listened to." So do all those ultra-romantic things, guys, but be a mensch, not a mouse.

Back to "Perpetual Courtship": "If a marriage is to be a compelling and continuing love story—and that's the goal here—romance must be reinvented, with new romantic challenges thrown in the way of the suitor (lawful husband though he be).

"The truth is, perpetual courtship is not an artificial contrivance, a trick foisted upon credulous husbands. It is an arrangement in harmony with our own biological natures, male and female. And even if it wasn't, who cares? It works!"

What's It All About, LFA? (9.3.08)

What's Wife Worship all about? Or any of its assorted alter egos and acronyms—Loving Female Authority (LFA), Female Led Relationships (FLR), and varieties of Marriages—Courtship,

Wife Led, Role Reversal and Matriarchal.

Is it all just an elaborate rationalization for off-kilter, slightly obsessive behavior, in bedroom and out? I mean, why write a whole book about it, or a blog that never ends?

Glad you asked. In response, I'll keep this post short and, I hope, sweet. And offer three concise answers from three people who practice and promote the Wife Worship lifestyle.

1) From an anonymously posting husband: "It's all about doing what I can do to make my wife happy. Because when she is happy, I'm happy. It doesn't take much once you get the hang of it. Every single day I just pretend we are dating and I try to win her heart."

2) From Emily Addison, co-author (with worshipful husband Ken) of the book, *Around Her Finger*, and the accompanying blog: "In last month's update [a] wife summed up the impact of loving female authority by saying that it simply made her feel loved. I think many women are loved by their husbands, but do not get enough validation to this effect...

"A woman whose husband respects her opinions, who works to please his wife, and who pampers her with foot massages and unselfish love-making—now that woman has few doubts. Women are very much creatures of our own emotions. When we can feel it, we know it is so."

3) From Katherine West, author of the "Loving Female Authority" blog: "I think the two key selling points for a woman are that first and foremost, [wife worship] is an expression of a man's love for his wife. Men have trouble expressing themselves. My husband's submission to me is love, just as my nurturing of his submission is also love.

"The second selling point is that it will make a woman's life more comfortable. He works hard to keep me happy. In doing so, it makes him happy. Incidentally, his happiness is not beside the point."

Comments:

Whatevershesays: You mean it's not about whips and chains? Thanks for compiling those summations. Important reading for the wives who think that it's just a sexual kink.

Mark: I know, it's vanilla-esque, and I get more commenters when I get edgier, but, hey, my wife reads this thing from time to time, and she's vanillaesque... and statuesque. And it is, after all, all about her.

Is Courtship Behavior a Fraud? (6.18.08)

An emailer objects to my passionate-courtship model for marriage:

"You're always advising husbands to act like they did when they were courting, which is already an old-fashioned concept, but that's phony behavior. Guys only do that stuff—buying flowers and candy and opening doors and even going to chick flicks—in order to get her to bed. Nobody actually lives like that. It's a fraud, part of the mating dance guys are supposed to go through."

Reading that reminded me of my dad, the way he once reacted to this European guy who would kiss ladies' hands on being introduced: "Phony hand-kissing," I remember my dad saying with contempt. "A real man saves that stuff for the bedroom."

I am also reminded of that ultimate anti-chivalric, chauvinist hero, Stanley Kowalski in Tennessee Williams' *Streetcar Named Desire*. Here's a famous exchange with Blanche DuBois: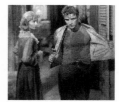

Blanche: I was fishing for a compliment, Stanley.
Stanley: I don't go in for that stuff.
Blanche: What?

Stanley: Compliments to women about their looks. I never met a dame yet that didn't know if she was good-looking or not without being told, and some of them give themselves credit for more than they've got. I once went out with a dame who told me, "I'm the glamorous type." She says, "I am the glamorous type!" I say, "So what?"

Blanche: And what did she say then?

Stanley: She didn't say nothing. That shut her up like a clam.

Blanche: Did it end the romance?

Stanley: Well, it ended the conversation, that was all. You know that some men, Blanche, that are took in by this Hollywood glamour stuff whereas some men just are not.

Blanche: I'm sure you belong in the second category.

Are these guys right, and I'm wrong? Should there be a post-nuptial ritual when husbands pull the pedestal out from under their new wives? Are male courtship rituals ridiculous and emasculating? Are they artificial and unsustainable?

I will agree that courtliness and chivalry are not easily sustained. Which is one reason so many marriages end unhappily. But is courtship behavior artificial? Let me quote my own book (Chapter 3, "Perpetual Courtship"):

"The truth is, perpetual courtship is not an artificial contrivance, a trick foisted upon credulous husbands. It is an arrangement in harmony with our own biological natures, male and female. And even if it wasn't, who cares? It works! What wife can hold out against continuous, insidious courtship? How can she not be susceptible?

"If a marriage is to be a compelling and continuing love story—and that's the goal here—romance must be reinvented, with new romantic challenges thrown in the way of the suitor (lawful husband though he be)."

Endlessly replaying the male-female mating dance is a secret a husband and wife can share, a little engine that can and could, that will generate erotic energy day after day.

It may not be the only secret to marital happiness. I haven't made a study, it's not my field. But it's certainly one secret, and I've seen many marriages collapse from its non-application.

The Kowalski Method may also seem like a workable formula for a sexually charged marriage, but unless the husband looks like the young Brando, I wouldn't advise him to try it.

Comments:

Susan's Pet: I see nothing wrong with ritual, protocol, courting, etc., as long as they are benign and get the job done. Many women, including my wife, are supportive of the hand-kissing Hollywood fakery, and they get off on it. Fine. If it does not cost you an arm and a leg, or a pair of balls, by all means do it. It makes her happy, which should in turn make you happy. It is not a matter of life or death. It is a matter of civility and refinement.

Mark: As another commenter said, some women don't like being put on a pedestal. In which case, you shouldn't keep hoisting 'em up there so you can worship them from below. But, as you say, courtship can proceed in terms of civility and refinement—and as a reminder to oneself that she is a prize beyond measure.

2

SAY HELLO TO YOUR QUEEN

Making *Her* Your Fantasy (6.9.08)

That's the title of Chapter 2 of my book. It's directed to husbands, and, of course, "her" refers to "wife." I could have said, "Making *Her* Your Fantasy — Again." The way she was during courtship, and the honeymoon. Until the glamour wore off somehow.

The point being, wives can regain that fantasy status. Because, to quote myself, "Men need sexual fantasy. It's the highest-octane fuel they can burn. They do idealize womanhood. They do empedestal their girlfriends."

Men are going to have those perpetual adolescent fantasies about some female or other. So shouldn't it be the woman we're married to, instead of Angelina Jolie or Scarlett Johansson or Jessica Simpson or whoever?

I know, guys think they can't control the sexual fantasy process. But, in fact, they can. If they want to, and are willing to make an effort for a glorious payoff.

The first step—stop masturbating. Easier preached than practiced, of course. I spent most of a chapter on the topic, and it's certainly more than I can deal with in this post. But, cutting to the chase, as I wrote...

"Once I stopped siphoning off the fuel needed for the marital combustion chambers, my sexual fantasies automatically refocused on my wife. She suddenly regained the status she possessed during courtship—seductress, enchantress. The creature to be pursued and won, again and again...

"I began thinking about her a lot. Daydreaming about her. Tripping out on tactile replays of her morning embrace, recalling the warm smell of her hair, the salty taste of her skin. She went, in the words of another song, from being 'gentle on my mind' to being very intrusive. In fact, I was thinking about her all the time. What I wasn't thinking about, or lusting after, were glamourized images of other females. Those had vaporized.'"

A commenter to this blog had the same experience when he stopped self-pleasuring. "Suddenly my wife looked really good to me," he wrote, "and I began what I could easily be called courting (I developed a crush on her—never thought I would feel that again)... Our sex life now is the best it has been since before we were married."

A dominant wife explains how it operates on her husband, referring to a photo of some glamorous actress: "I have to admit, girls, this young and beautiful woman on the left is what I would like to look like. Once a long, long time ago, I kinda looked like her, but even in my 20s, I didn't look as good. Now, I'm in my 50s and gravity is winning more and more every day. But in the eyes and mind of my husband, I am FAR, FAR, superior to this beautiful young lady, because to him I am his Goddess and his Queen, I am beautiful in his mind and eyes and he shows it to me EVERY Minute of EVERY day."

Once this begins happening to a husband, he can actively encourage the process, and he will find himself living with a fantasy figure.

Or, to quote my favorite bit of advice on this topic, "If you want your wife to be a goddess, worship her."

Comments:

Burnsie: I can tell you for a fact that quitting masturbation does indeed work. My wife and I have been together for 19 years, and since I stopped (and got rid of all the porn) our sex life has been the best. The teasing, the flirting, the cuddling, the orgasms! WOW!

Yes, I did get rid of all porn, electronic and paper. I deleted all book-marks, broke all CDs in half, and recycled all the magazines. I bet the recycling guys loved to find those mags in the bin.

Mark: Been there, done that. In fact, embarrassingly enough, more than once! I once codified this precept: "Unshared pleasures become private vices." It certainly holds true for me.

There must be millions of these collections squirreled away on hard disks, flash drives, CDs, etc., now that porn of every stripe is so easily available online. And I had my share...

Now, I confess, I still have a small collection of images that glorify femi-ninity that I use for the blog, but which I need not hide from my wife. In fact, I want her to know how much I worship the female form, first and foremost hers!

Burnsie: My wife commented that we have been having more and better sex over the past two months than we have had over the past several years. I told her that I haven't been looking at any porn for almost three months. That I got rid of all of it. That she is the only woman that I desire and fantasize about. The smile I got from her was priceless!

Becoming President of Her Fan Club (4.10.08)

Are you the president of your wife's fan club? Is she the radiant center of your universe? Does she leave you star-struck, blinded by her luminescence? Do you, like ardent Curly in *Oklahoma!* collect treasured keepsakes from your beloved? ("Give me back my rose and my glove.")

If this sounds romantically retarded, give it another think. Didn't you once feel that way about her? Star-struck and lovestruck? When you were courting? So, in keeping with the perpetual courtship marriage, the kind of FLR I advocate in my book, why not act that way again?

A co-worker once told me about this sexy new temp in his office, a Latina bombshell who turned him into Jello. When she agreed to go out with him, he went binge-shopping—for chocolates (Godiva), roses (two dozen red). When he'd called to ask her out, he'd even asked what her favorite perfume was and bought some of that, at like $40 an ounce (this was twenty years ago). The guy just couldn't help himself.

"I don't care if I go overboard," he told me. "You know what Alicia told me on the phone? She gives this incredible throaty chuckle and tells me, 'Oh, you're going to be wonderful for my ego!'"

What higher compliment could a girl give her fan club president?

This story reminds me of another, a reminiscence by the famous Hollywood actor, Robert Taylor. He wasn't famous, though, when he was cast opposite the great Greta Garbo in *Camille*. Handsome, yes, but almost unknown, and not much of an actor, to be candid. But Garbo liked his princely looks and got him the part. Then proceeded 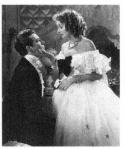 to cast her spell over him, exactly as her character, Marguerite Gautier, does to his character, Armand Duval, in the film.

During the course of filming, Taylor spent hours in her dressing room as her enchanted captive, listening to her husky voice, looking at the memorabilia of her fabulous career, hopelessly intoxicated with her. And Garbo not only seduced Taylor, but induced from the too-laid-back actor a compelling performance. It comes across on screen—but, of course, he wasn't acting. He was madly in love.

Alas, when filming wrapped, Garbo dismissed him completely. But he had been, at least for magical moment in time, the president of her fan club.

My turn to confide. I was a ninth-grader in a high school art class, seated by blessed fate in the back row next to a glamorous senior girl, a regal beauty whom I will call LaDonna Dillon. She had, like that, a camera-ready name. She starred in school plays—in sophisticated, decadent Tennessee Williams' plays, believe it or not. Like *Orpheus Descending*. In high school! She spoke in a theatrical whisper. She was magnificent. And I guess she thought I was... well, kind of cute, with my goggle glasses and crewcut and obvious puppypdog adoration of her.

One morning I arrived early at the art bungalow and found LaDonna there, alone, working on a project. I took my place next to her and opened a book on Renoir, the artist I'd chosen for my book report. Next thing I knew, LaDonna had scooted her stool closer, was right there, a perfumed erotically charged presence, looking over my shoulder at Renoir's succulent nudes. In fact, at one point LaDonna reached over my shoulder and began turning pages, asking me which ones I liked best. My head was spinning, and that was the least of my organic reactions!

I was ready to establish the LaDonna Dillon Fan Club and Goddess Worship Society right then and there. (As it was, she went on to have a minor Hollywood career without me, mostly in episodic TV.)

Let me exit from this overlong post with a quote from one of my wife-worship role models, Au876, who posted for several years on Lady Misato's original Wife Worship forum. Here's his encouraging advice on becoming your wife's number-one fan:

"Never miss a chance to tell her how beautiful she is, how smart she is and how much you cherish her. Rub her feet at night. Give her pedicures, fold her night gown, clean her hair brush (daily), rub her back, tend her bath (for example a simple thing like bringing her a hot towel to dry off with is little trouble and yet very sweet)... Let your adoration spill over."

Amen, Au. Rah! Rah! Rah!

SAY HELLO TO YOUR QUEEN

Living With a Goddess (7.1.08)

"The deadening scales of familiarity will dissolve, and you will see her restored to full, feminine mystery and radiance."— *Worshipping Your Wife*, Chapter 3, "Making Her Your Fantasy"

It's a visionary experience almost to die for, and definitely to live for, one which will forever transform your marriage and your life.

What does it feel like to live with a goddess on a daily basis? I'll let these wife-worshipping husbands supply their own giddy responses:

"A wave of profound happiness rises in me when I worship my Goddess wife. It is heaven for me."

"Through my wife I am brought close to the center of the feminine mystery, intoxicated by it, overwhelmed by her."

"[My wife] has arrived home and my heart is fluttering with excitement! I do not feel complete until she is home. I'm an intimate part of the life of a beautiful woman. So close to her, caring only for her comfort and happiness...

"I have just hung her silk suit in her closet when, whap! Her panties hit me in the face and she laughs playfully. I put them in my hand-wash basket and turn to gaze adoringly at my Mistress.

"Naked, stretching her beautiful body, absolutely comfortable in front of me, she turns her brilliant emerald eyes on me and smiles, knowing exactly what effect she is having on me and enjoying it...

"As she strides past me, all energy, grace and unselfconscious nakedness, she slaps my ass hard and, to her amusement, I squeal and jump and hurry to do her bidding."

"I love to wash my wife's hair and scrub her in the shower, then dry her. She loves it too. If someone says it isn't important, I do not care. I know giving and loving are important to me."

"My wife makes me worship her, pray to her and chant to her. Sexual service is a part of my ritual in worshipping her. It is a beautiful thing. I humble myself before my wife and pray to her. Then I kiss her feet and slowly work my worshipful kisses up

31

her legs and eventually make my way to her shrine, the place where all life begins. Once there, I worship her by licking her to orgasm while she chants a lovely song about the superiority of women in her sexy and hypnotic voice. I feel so at peace and nurtured by her, as I taste of her. It is not uncommon for both my wife and I to have tears in our eyes during this sacred ritual."

Comments:
Anonymous: This is a beautiful narration of a goddess-worship ritual. It is so true in front of women we men are nothing. It is only a woman's generosity that she allows a male to worship her body, her femininity. Women are no less than goddesses. We should fulfill all of their desires without any inhibitions.

Swagger vs. Grovel, Part 1 (12.21.07)

A primal response of a young male on encountering a beautiful female may be to strut and swagger, but another, and perhaps even more primal response is to be awestruck.

Hollywood movies, notably westerns and action-adventures, have celebrated the taciturn, macho hero—Cooper and Peck, Wayne and McQueen, Eastwood and Bronson, Costner and Stallone. Marlon Brando embodied this tomcat nonchalance as Stanley Kowalski in *Streetcar*:

Blanche DuBois: "I was fishing for a compliment."
Stanley Kowalski: "I don't go in for that stuff."

But another masculine archetype has been on wide-screen display in Hollywood comedies. Here you find grown men reduced to stammering, groveling adolescence by mere proximity to female splendor. Take your pick: Tom Ewell with Marilyn Monroe in *Seven Year Itch*, Tony Randall with Jayne Mansfield in *Will Success Spoil Rock Hunter?*, Jack Lemmon with Monroe and Kim Novak and other bombshell beauties in any number of comedies.

Male inadequacy is front and center, of course, in the nerdy film personas of Jerry Lewis and Woody Allen. A perfect example can be seen in a YouTube clip from *Hollywood or Bust*, which shows Jerry Lewis literally falling head over heels at sight of Anita Ekberg.

The geek-and-goddess romance becomes thematic with Dudley Moore, who was *Bedazzled* by Raquel Welch and bewitched by Bo Derek in *10*. In the original *Heartbreak Kid*, screenwriter Neil Simon has buttoned-down honeymooner Charles Grodin up and dump his Brooklynesque bride to pursue the Minnesota shiksa perfection of Cybill Shepherd.

But it's not just nerds and geeks who willingly succumb to the power of female sexuality. Check out any strip club in a blue-collar neighborhood (where many tend to be), especially on a local payday, and you'll see truck drivers, factory workers, mechanics and Hell's Angel wannabes packed shoulder to shoulder in the stage-side seats, gaping up in idolatrous awe and hanging their hard-earned cash along the railing. These are offerings to the prancing priestesses on high, who do the strutting and swaggering, affording the acolytes below only sneak peeks into forbidden paradise.

Goddess worship could hardly be more explicit, nor the imbalance of power between male supplicant and dominant female more visible. *Vive la différence!*

Comments:
Unknown Alien: I very much connect to your description to this reaction to a beautiful woman as that of awe. I feel that the source of this awe is in fact something exceedingly commanding, powerful and conquering.
Mark: Dear UA, this awestruck response is the jumping-off place in my own experience for all this wife-worship stuff. I can't control the response, and it can be almost overpowering, like being swept with some kind of brain-overload, however you want to describe it, even religious ecstasy.

Swagger vs. Grovel, Part 2 (10.20.09)

One of the early posts on this blog, back in December 2007, was titled "Swagger vs Grovel." It contrasted two "primal" male responses on encountering a beautiful female:

1. to strut and swagger, or
2. to be awestruck

As examples of "first responders," I listed some familiar icons of movie masculinity—John Wayne, Clint Eastwood, Charles Bronson, *et al.*

But, guess what, just as many popular Hollywood actors can be found in the second category of responders—"men reduced to stammering, groveling adolescence by mere proximity to female splendor." I cited Jerry Lewis, Woody Allen, Jack Lemmon and many others, including, prototypically, Dudley Moore in *10*.

One among many groveling leading guys whom I overlooked, a familiar face on vintage movie channels, is Danny Kaye, especially in his Walter Mittyesque pursuit of Virginia Mayo.

In these films, I noted, "goddess worship could hardly be more explicit, nor the imbalance of power between male supplicant and dominant female more visible."

I fancied my "swagger vs. grovel" formulation rather original. But I am not unhappy to learn that others have explored these same ideas and, in at last once instance, penetrated far deeper into the matter. In fact, it has prompted this sequel to that two-year-old posting.

I have in mind a short article on male psychology, "What Are You Staring At?" by Tomomi Kumakura, Ph.D. It can be found reprinted on the Dreamlover Labs website among their "Male Management" articles. I don't know the original publication source.

In the article's opening paragraphs the "swagger" response is defined as "active lust," and "grovel" as "passive lust:

"There are two psychologically distinct ways in which males can perceive a woman's beauty... The first psychological stance is that of the predator. In this case, the male's arousal is accompanied by what I call 'active lust' which can be summed up as a wish to dominate the female and make her his through copulation.

"The second possible stance that males can have is, however, a lot more interesting... and it consists in the same intense arousal associated with a sensation of worshipfulness, reverence, adoration; sometimes even awe. I call this 'passive lust.'"

The writer goes on to explain how this type of lust renders husbands and boyfriends much more amenable to behavior modification by the women in their lives:

"The 'worshipful trance' of the drooling, seduced male is a desired state in which willful compliance can be obtained; in fact, the ease of training of most naturally compliant males derives from the psychological position of weakness they perceive when exposed to feminine beauty... This sort of male is 'locked into' the passive lust modality."

The article continues in a similar tongue-in-cheek behavioristic vein, yet, despite her playfulness, I don't think Dr. Kumakura can be written off as a mere parodist, even when she explains how she exploits her own husband's passive lust on her own behalf. Her psychological observations on this topic ring absolutely true to me—and I should know.

As I wrote to one who commented on my first "Swagger vs. Grovel" posting, "[A sense of awe and worshipfulness when faced with feminine beauty] is the jumping-off place in my own experience for all this wife-worship stuff. I can't control the response, and it can be almost overpowering, like being swept with some kind of brain-overload, however you want to describe it, even religious ecstasy."

Hey, but isn't that how Rocky Balboa felt about Adrian? Be careful, you macho guys. It could happen to you.

Comments:

Anonymous WLM Couple: Passive lust is what I experience as my wife likes to tease me often. I must face the wall if she wishes to change clothes while in the bedroom. When she exits the shower she will call to me when her towel is wrapped around her so that I may come in and dry down the entire shower area. My wife feels that all of this visual denial keeps me more interested and in a state of arousal, and it does. All of this, combined with her denying me orgasms for long periods, keeps me in a state of passive lust.

Isn't She Simply Divine? Part 1 (8.8.08)

As I said in my book (Chapter 5, Page 48): "Worshipping Your Wife is not about literal worship (goddess or otherwise), idolatry or anything even remotely sacrilegious. It is about respecting and honoring, revering and protecting, adoring and cherishing."

I went on to belabor the obvious point: "We're speaking poetically—the hyperbolic language of lovestruck suitors. It is through this rose-colored prism we view the creatures we love. 'All women are goddesses,' screen goddess Nicole Kidman decreed... Boyfriends need to understand that if women are worshiped, the world will be a better place.'"

Issue settled? You might think so, but you'd be wrong. Some newcomers attracted to the wonderful world of Female-Led Relationships are ready to do a 180 when they encounter the "Worship" word.

Like this guy: "As much as I love my bride, I cannot, will not, put her in the place of God in my life, and as such can't consider 'wife worship.' The *Bible* says that we are to worship God alone (*Revelations* 19:10 and 22:9). And if I attempt to put anybody or anything in God's place, my life falls apart."

I certainly don't intend to offend anyone's faith, or launch a debate on Biblical exegesis and theology. I thought I was dealing in romantic metaphor, the "hyperbolic language of love," using "worship" figuratively, as a daily and reverential attitude that combines love and devotion, honoring and cherishing.

But maybe that's not clear enough. So I've dredged up a few responses to this objection.

Here's one from Fumika Misato's original Wife Worship Ya-hoo Forum (back in 1999) from a poster screen-named "pbear": "[My wife] suggested that wife worship was sacreligious and it made her uncomfortable. I worship God and thank God for bringing my wife into my life and pray that I am given the strength to stay focused on her and the role she plays in my life."

Lady Misato offered her own clarification: "I don't think that anyone's use of the term 'worship,' including myself, means anything of a religious level. And I'm not sure how serious even the most serious female-supremacists are about the religious content. At best, they are more spiritually oriented."

"I agree with Lady Misato," amened Au876. "We are talking about submitting to our wife, putting her needs and wants above our on... We are not praying to her and while we may be seek-ing her guidance, we don't think it is divine."

Or, as I wrote in an earlier blog-post: "We intend no sacri-lege; I think we just get carried away."

But this does not close the case. Some worshipful husbands, and worshipped wives *do* use the "W" verb non-poetically, it seems. "My wife has started referring to herself as goddess," writes a devout husband, "and I've tried to treat her like one, even to the point of worship. She has no problem whatsoever with my 'idolatry.'"

Years ago a young man sought Elise Sutton's advice when his girlfriend made the same demand: "My girlfriend wants me to literally worship her as a Superior Being, a Goddess if you will, in both physical and psychological aspects. However, I am hav-ing trouble with this request. Wouldn't I be guilty of idolatry in the physical act of worshipping my Mistress? My girlfriend is a staunch believer in female supremacy and says that it is okay for me to worship God's most perfect creatures on earth."

Elise's response resonates with Lady Misato's: "Your girlfriend is challenging you to explore the spiritual aspects of the female domination lifestyle. I am sure she does not feel she is a deity. It sounds like she wants you to recognize her superiority over you and she is demanding that you worship her as your earthly Goddess."

But Ms. Sutton is only getting started on this provocative topic: "It is a beautiful thing when a man humbles himself before a woman and worships her as his earthly Goddess. Humility is an important aspect of Christianity. Jesus humbled himself before his disciples as he washed their feet during the last supper. Was he committing idolatry? No, he was serving them and teaching them how to serve one another… When you bow before your superior Goddess, you are recognizing her supreme position over you. You are not exalting her above God. If you did that, then you would be committing idolatry. But if you exalt her as your earthly Queen and Goddess, you should be able to rectify that with your conscience."

Then Ms. Sutton goes a step farther on the issue of idolatry. There are female supremacists who encourage, and even demand what she believes is idolatrous worship from their men:

"I know some women who actually make their submissive men pray to them. They make them perform rituals as they worship their earthly Goddess. I have never embraced that sort of female domination due to my conscience…"

I was aware of that, of course, when I wrote the book, but chose not to delve too deeply into such practices. But perhaps I will in another post, Part 2 of "Isn't She Simply Divine?"

Comments:
Anonymous: I have put my Wife in a "divine position" in my life, and I recognize that completely. (She doesn't necessarily care how I rationalize it to myself, as long as I obey.) I'm not a believer in any kind of Celestial Deity, and as long as I have Her, I don't feel the need for one. I am fully aware that she's not "a goddess" in the "Omnipotent Creator" sense, but I deify her in the following ways:

1. I assume she can see my soul, therefore she would know instantly if I were to lie or in any way be untrue to her.

2. "Blind Faith." I take her word as Gospel. I unquestioningly do as she says and accept what she tells me as Truth. Like many religious people, I take her word over "facts" or doubt.

3. Because she is a superior being, Rules don't apply to Her, at least not as far as we are concerned. She can do no wrong, and has "Divine Infallibility."

4. I do, at times, formally Worship her. I don't pray as in asking for things. It usually will consist of her sitting or lying down while I kneel and spout Devotions to Her.

I don't recommend giving such faith in just anyone, it has taken years to build that kind of trust to put such devotion in a human being. She doesn't insist I do any of this, I consider it an honor that she allows me to. I also don't expect her to be perfect. Sometimes I show my devotion by freely giving her a shoulder to cry on or offering advice. Whatever She needs of me.

I feel that many people in search of God are really searching for Unconditional Love, Forgiveness and Acceptance. These are all things I find with Her.

Mark: Anonymous, what you say resonates with me, because I have had a lifelong problem with worship, though I am a believer. But all my worshipful emotions are instantly accessible when I view God's most sublime creation—and I am happy that my wife has now assumed that exalted place in my life. I am coming to grips with this, or trying to, in these postings.

Isn't She Simply Divine? Part 2 (8.11.08)

In Part 1 of this post (and in my book) I explained that "Worshipping Your Wife is not about literal worship (goddess or otherwise), idolatry or anything even remotely sacrilegious. It is about respecting and honoring, revering and protecting, adoring and cherishing."

But that's not the whole story. As I pointed out on my original website, "In some female-supremacist organizations, males do literally worship females; and in coupled relationships, literally worship their partners (by whatever agreed-upon exalted title). In some instances, there are even religious trappings—thrones and altars and confessions and so forth."

WORSHIPPING YOUR WIFE 2

To these couples, of course, such worship does not constitute idolatry, as the wife is viewed as an embodiment of the Goddess.

One of the longest-running Goddess-worshipping organizations that I'm aware of is the Service of Mankind Church, active since the late '70s in the S.F. Bay Area. Also known as the "SM Church," "Essemian (ess-EM-ian) Church" or "Church of the "Surrendered Male," the organization worships the "Darkside Goddess (Kali)," who is usually shown with her foot on the prostrate corpse of the male deity Shiva.

According to one of the Church websites, "A growing number of special women, some wearing long, flowing robes and capes, and thonged sandals upon their feet, others clad all in leather, spike-heeled shoes or boots, and carrying implements of bondage or punishment, are being called 'goddesses' and worshipped by those who humbly bow their heads to the floor at their feet... The *Essemian Manifesto* describes in religious philosophical terms the postulation that certain acts of female dominance, when ritualized as psychodrama, can be a religious experience."

If the Essemians represent the dark side of goddess worship, Rasa von Werder emphasizes a blinding white luminescence on her web pages and in her matriarchal "Mother of God Church."

Like the Essemians, Ms. Von Werder has been around a while, having achieved a certain fame in decades past as a female bodybuilder, stripper and Playboy's Miss Nude Universe under the name of Kellie Everts. Ms. Von Werder, in fact, maintains a separate "Kellie Everts, Stripper for God" website.

How can any church not similarly endowed compete with that? Ms. Everts/Von Werder must get rather a lot of applications from new enthusiastic male converts.

I didn't delve deeply enough into her abundant offerings to see if she encourages her devotees to build an altar to worship her, but other Goddess organizations have made this a prerequisite to advanced study, as in this admonition from the "Femina Society" (apparently no longer Googleable): "Student initiates must erect an Alcove (Altar) of Respect with one or more of Her

40

artifacts (inquire) or a Goddess figurine of Her choice."

This may sound wildly kinky and fetishistic. But is endowing some innocent artifact with Goddess-like powers really so different from some common courtship behaviors, like the one amusingly described in *Oklahoma!* by the lovely Laurey in "People Will Say We're in Love"?

She warns her boyfriend Curly (in Hammerstein's lyrics):

Don't start collecting things
Give me my rose and my glove.
Sweetheart, they're suspecting things
People will say we're in love.

Was Curly accumulating fetish objects for his private altar to Laurey?

Maybe. But here are two unarguable examples of idolatry-at-home, both from letters to the invaluable Elise Sutton "Female Superiority" website:

1. "My wife makes me worship her, pray to her and chant to her. Sexual service is a part of his ritual in worshipping her. It is a beautiful thing. I humble myself before my wife and pray to her. Then I kiss her feet and slowly work my worshipful kisses up her legs and eventually make my way to her shrine, the place where all life begins. Once there, I worship her by licking her to orgasm while my wife chants a lovely song about the superiority of women in her sexy and hypnotic voice. I feel so at peace and nurtured by her, as I taste of her. It is not uncommon for both me and my wife to have tears in our eyes during this sacred ritual."

2. "My Mother was a staunch Female Supremacist and lived it 365/24/7. It was her lifestyle and her religion. She was a Goddess, and she knew it... My father had to worship her as his earthly Goddess and be her slave. My Mother had ceremonies and rituals where the men had to worship the women."

In each of these instances, the apotheosis was initiated by the woman, but more often the impetus comes from the male acolyte, who wants to exalt his wife into a goddess. A typical plea:

41

"Is it wrong for me to worship beautiful women? Is it normal for me to create an elaborate altar that idolizes beautiful women? This is what is in my heart! To me, it is about serving a living deity. Am I the only male who feels this way?"

Absolutely not. I'll confess, I'm another such. And what about this guy, who clearly harbors the self-same worshipful yearning:

"I would like my wife to assert her true female goddess identity and let me openly worship her the way I have to do in private now. I would welcome the worshipping lifestyle in ways in which would I'm sure would make my wife's life heavenly."

But let me back up to that earlier question to Elise —"Is it wrong for me to worship beautiful women?" Her answer begins with a theological clarification: "The practice of exalting people, animals, and nature above God is known as idolatry and if you are Jewish or a Christian, idolatry is the violation of the very first commandment. ('You shall have no other Gods before Me'). The key words are 'before me,' so you can worship women, but be careful not to replace the Creator with the creation. Women were created to be served by men and to govern men from a position of authority. Women were not created to replace God in men's lives."

After lecturing the man, she gives him a maternal pat on the head: "I can fully understand your desire to want to worship women in a deeper and more spiritual way… Women are worthy to be worshipped but you must be careful to worship women in a manner that will meet their practical needs. Building an altar and meditating on the beauty and majesty of women might be good for you personally, and thus be mentally and spiritually satisfying, but it has no practical benefit to women."

Grab a mop and a broom, in other words. Clean the altar and the holy ground all around. And then ask your Goddess what else She'd like done.

Here's a wife who obviously is worshipped in exactly that way: "Dear Elise, My husband has learned to obey me and, indeed, to worship me, and I truly believe that he is a better person for the experience."

I'm not attempting a conclusion here, just a survey of a provocative field. But, if a conclusion needs to be reached, let's have Elise Sutton do the summing up, in her best counseling voice:

"Do you feel guilty about worshipping your wife and serving her as her slave? This is merely an advanced form of romance and intimacy. Don't make too much out of the word 'worship.' Religion elevates these words to unattainable standards when they really talk to our most basic nature. You love God so you sing songs of praise and you worship God. You love your wife so you adore her, praise her and show her acts of devotion. It is not the same kind of worship because your wife is flesh and blood whereas God is Spirit but they both involve intimacy. Worship is an act of intimacy."

Comments:
Norman: Females are more divine than are males. God made Women, and appointed us to serve and worship them. The females need answer to no one but God. If we worship our female above all others, knowing She is subservient to God only, then aren't we fulfilling the Commandment by proxy?
Mark: It works for me!

Fuller Is Better (4.28.08)

"Our devotion to our wonderful wives doesn't come with dress-size limits."— pseudonymous wife-worshipper

It's true, dear wives, so true! We worship you "just the way you are," as Billy Joel famously sang.

As I remind husbands in my book (Chapter 2, "Making Her Your Fantasy," p. 18-19): "…this is another gift you can give your wife: Be adoring, be accepting, be the safe haven where she can be totally and comfortably herself. Because you accept her just the way she is, it's easier for her to accept herself. This can have a healing effect on her psyche—particularly if she's dissatisfied with her body or her looks—and provide a well-deserved boost for her ego."

Alas, too many women are dissatisfied with their looks (in fact, a majority of them, according to surveys), and too many strive to be shed pounds and curves that only enhance their desirability in the eyes of their worshipful husbands.

But here's one woman who profoundly gets it, female supremacist Paige Harrison. She writes on her website: "My husband absolutely loves my body. He worships my goddess belly, savors my round bottom, and adores my big breasts and full thighs. Also, my hips look great in a tight pair of jeans... I am a big girl now and love it and feel fantastic about my size 14/16 body."

This husband emphatically agrees: "I do truly love my wife's rounder figure, fuller breasts and more shapely behind. In my view, fuller is better, and these skeletons that are supposed to represent fashion are on the way out. The Dove ads teach us to accept all women in all of their glorious manifestations, and I think that is a valuable lesson to all of us males."

Let me give the last word to a former wife-worshipping blog-colleague, "fdhousehusband," who writes:

"It is funny how my taste in Womyn has matured over the years. There was a time when i was so much taken with society's vision of perfect, thin Womyn. Yet, over the years, as my Wife has enjoyed the fruits of Her career success, She has put on some weight and now would be considered to be overweight by society. To me, however, my Wife seems more Beautiful than ever and i find myself being turned on more and more by such Rubenesque Womyn."

Comments:
Fd: Yes, "fuller is better" in many ways. i feel that my Wife is now free from the bonds of society that dictates that Womyn should starve themselves.

my Wife is happy with Who She is and that is the sexiest thing in the world.

EF: As far back as my first girlfriend in 6th grade, I've loved full-figured women. My wife is one, and I find her to be the sexiest and most attractive woman I've ever seen. It's sad that she is not so accepting of her own body.

Mark: EF, it is exactly my situation and sentiment. If only she could see herself as I see her—and I'm trying my utmost to convey to her how beauteous she is to behold.

Her Cups Runneth Over (9.26.08)

Let me briefly belabor the obvious. The size and shape, let alone touch and taste, of a beauteous female breast reverts most men into instant baby boyhood. Abracadabra-fast.

If it wasn't considered Neanderthal behavior and a major social no-no, we'd get whiplashed by every passing rack. And if no one's looking, we do. It's never easy or natural not to.

Ask Madison Avenue. Ask Hollywood. Ask any woman, of even modest endowment. If a glimpse of stocking used to be considered shocking, what of the effect on men of today's ubiquitous push-em-up cleavage? Well, it tends to putty the masculine will, jelly the knees and spine, while stiffening elsewhere.

Talk about power exchange! Maternal, matriarchal, whatever you call it, it's irresistible!

Most women in female-led relationships fully realize this, of course, and take full advantage. Some leading wives, I read, severely restrict their husband's access to their breasts, except as a rare reward for exceptional devotion and service.

Other women, I'm happy to report, take the opposite tack, allowing their males regular intervals of prolonged breast worship, with apparently delightful consequences to both parties.

It is these more generous souls, sharers of the mammary wealth I choose to quote here, rather than the off-limiting wives.

"I don't allow my husband to fondle, kiss, or lick my breasts," writes one such wife. "I *make* him do it! I enjoy it very much! So therefore. I have him pay attention to them for as long as I want or until it's time for me to have him go onto the next thing."

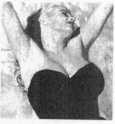

"I always start out by allowing my husband to plant passionate kisses all over my body." writes another sharing wife. "He starts at my feet and works up my body. It is when his body worship finally reaches my abundant breasts that whatever was on his mind will vanish and he becomes lost in my world and I know that I have him in the palms of my hands."

Another: "I love having my breasts sucked and nibbled on and I have been known to make him perform breast worship for over an hour at a time. I call it tit worship, as that sounds sexier."

And here's another lucky suckler: "When I was about 20, I had a lovely girlfriend of similar age. I would suckle her beautiful breasts for long stretches of time in accordance with her instructions. Mothering became so important in our lives that she would have me suckle even when she wasn't in the mood to have sex."

Psychologist Paige Harrison prescribes regular sessions of this kind of bosom-bonding to the female-led couples she counsels: "A refreshingly different perspective can be experienced if the male understands it his responsibility to worship the female whenever her breasts are exposed. If she exposes her breasts, this should have a calming effect on the submissive male."

"Something new I have introduced into our female-led lifestyle," says yet another sharing spouse. "After my husband undresses me I unhook the cups and allow him to suck while I hold him for extended periods of time. He really seems to appreciate this. Afterward he seems to be much more attentive to my needs and feelings."

I'll give the last word to a husband whose wife used nursing sessions as a kind of confessional therapy for him: "Sometimes I do things I should not do and when I began confessing these transgressions to my wife, at first I was a bit bashful, stuttering a little. She instinctively pulled me close to her chest, my face nuzzled between her breasts. I felt so safe and secure in her embrace.

"Then she unbuttoned her blouse and proceeded to nurse me from her breasts. She said, 'It's OK, honey, I'm glad you were honest with me. I just want you to think about it when you sleep.' There was this overwhelming sense of childlike security, being near her breasts, feeling pure and forgiven. I loved how she gently stroked my hair while watching me nurse."

Where's my binky?

Comments:

Jboy: The bosom of a dominant woman controlling an FLR symbolizes her role as the ultimate provider of love, leadership and security to her family. All are dependant upon her and surrender themselves to her authority for she is capable of leading and controlling their lives. Though her children will be set free in adulthood, Her hubby will go deeper under Her control and belong entirely to his loving Wife.

Mark: I particularly like your final line, jboy, about her children being set free in adulthood and hubby going "deeper under her control." My hope exactly!

Burnsie: My wife read this article and loved it. I see more of her breasts now. After she's been working out or doing something that makes her sweaty she takes off her top and tells me to lick the sweat from her breasts. Other times I just have to sit there and look at them and she teases me with them.

Anonymous: My gorgeous, 6'1" man—a college professor with a doctorate—nurses at my breasts every day. My breasts are quite large as they are producing amounts that he wants. He came to America at age 11, but had lived in a remote part of Sicily and was breastfed until the age of 5. He takes milk from each breast for about 15 minutes, and it arouses me to a point of orgasm. I don't know if any other couples do this, but what one does in private is our own business—and we both love it.

Mark: Anonymous, you win the award for hot comment of the year, no contest. Be still my beating heart! I join with all my male readers in envying your well-nursed husband, a most happy fella, I'm sure. Thanks for sharing with us... but then, we already knew you were a generous lady!

Anonymous: I worship my wife's "Rack of Ages" and nursed on them long after each child was born! She loves to go around the house almost topless and wishes more women would read your article. She definitely does not need for the Lord to fill her cups for they are already full enough!

Mark: Are you married to the Anonymous wife who posted 2 posts above you? If not, perhaps I've tapped into a provocative trend among worshipful husbands and their well-endowed wives. It's sounding like an afternoon TV topic—and one I would certainly tune in on! Lucky you!

Anonymous: No, I'm not married to her. It does not surprise me that both of our teenage boys have rather buxom girlfriends. On Valentine's Day my wife let me lick chocolate body paint she had bought for us off of her breasts. Wow, that was one powerful sexual experience.

Bow and Vow (11.29.08)

Nothing to do with *Worshipping Your Wife*, even the occasional royalty, makes me happier than getting emails from readers about how my book or blog helped advance their female-led relationships. Not always, but usually it is men who confide that my prescriptions actually helped or, even better, that they showed certain chapters or blog posts to the potential goddess in their life, and she took the wife worship message to heart!

One gracious reader, in a recent series of email exchanges, credited my writings for "giving me the courage to openly submit to my wonderful wife." After a period of "stealth submission," he "came out" to his recent bride with a letter "explaining everything."

Submissive hubbies who have gone the stealth submission route well know the anxiety involved in such a "coming out," finding the right confessional tone and words, then waiting like a prisoner in the dock for the reaction of the beloved, searching her face and body language for the first signs of yea or nay.

My email correspondent hit the jackpot. His bride's reaction to his confessional letter was everything he had hoped and prayed for. "She thought it was beautiful," he wrote. Later he showed his wife my book, and she was enthusiastic. My friend is now living a life of open submission, and has since shared my book with another man. He adds, "I am beyond happy."

He provides some additional details that I'd like to share. Every day he gets down on his knees and affirms his adoration of his beloved. "I honestly don't remember the first time I knelt in front of her and just adored her," he writes. It just seemed natural. Down on his knees he repeats a series of daily vows that he wrote. "I say these to her every day, no exceptions."

Here they are, minus a few personal phrases. I find them romantic and tender, candid and, yes, intimately confessional:

Today I promise to show you my love in how I speak to you and listen to you.

Today I promise to treat you with affection and respect.

Today I promise to put your needs before my needs and your desires before my desires.

You are my wife, my lover, my fantasy and my queen and I very much want to please you.

I very much want to serve and obey you.

I want to belong to you. I want to be your submissive husband.

This is who I am and I adore you for accepting me.

This daily ritual serves as a reminder of and rededication to his life of submissive devotion to his wife. And, he writes, borrowing a phrase from my book, it is also part of "daring to be known by her."

I felt a pang of jealousy when I read this, because my new friend was describing a ritual that I once practiced with my wife, but which several years ago I allowed to slip away through lack of conviction and commitment to the lifestyle. As I explained in my own note to my wife:

"When I see you each morning, or at the end of each workday, my heart fills with a newlywed's happiness. But, after 13 years of marriage [note: that was 8 years ago], there is no accepted ritual that permits me to display the intensity of my feelings. So I make do with a casual peck, a squeeze, a touch in passing... Too many months ago, for a brave while, I dared to go farther—to steal a few seconds out of our hectic morning preparations to kneel before you, as you dressed or did your makeup, and to embrace you wholeheartedly and declare my devotion. You were, I recall, accepting of these awkward avowals, and they gave my spirits a euphoric lift, a sense of going into the day draped with milady's colors and enwrapped in milady's perfume... But I let them lapse. And though I miss them keenly, these giddy little rituals, I've been too embarrassed, or too timid, to attempt to renew them."

And here my new email friend, inspired by me, was enjoying this wonderful daily ritual which I had neglected and lost! Why did I let that happen? I made my own vow—to regain what I had lost. To refresh my memory, I did a quick search of some postings I had saved on the topic of daily vows and obeisances. Here are a couple that get to the heart of the matter:

"When [my wife] finally got out of bed I quickly assumed my morning place before Her, kneeling before her, kissing her feet while she sat on the edge of the bed. She allowed this daily morning obeisance for a few moments, then stood and walked away toward her bathroom."

Even more to the point is this posting from the wonderful blog (linked on my home page) by "Mistress Kathy" known as "Femdom 101":

"One of the special moments in my life was the first time John knelt at my feet, and we talked as mistress and [husband]. In my view the first time a man has the courage to kneel at his wife's feet is a very special occasion. This special little physical act often helps a couple transcend many of the boundaries that have kept their marriage arrangement from moving forward.

"This may seem strange to many of you, but that moment John knelt to me for the first time, was as much of a romantic occasion as our first kiss. [Now, five years later] there is never a day that John does not get down on his knees in front of me. During that time we talk as husband and wife, and John gives me his full and complete attention. There are no cell phones, TV, or other interruptions allowed. Our talk always ends with a kiss when I give him permission to rise.

"What I am hoping… is to encourage other aspiring couples to adopt this procedure into their lives. It would make me very happy if at least one couple, who tries this procedure, would give me their comments on how this simple little act of devotion made them feel. I would love to hear as much from the wife as the husband."

So thank you to my email correspondent. I am rewarded to have inspired you. But now you have inspired me. I make a bow and vow today to regain that wonderful daily ritual, which began for me years ago as an impulsive hyper-romantic gesture. I will keep you posted, and Mistress Kathy, too, on how I do in following through.

Comments:
Bob: I love to read about the romantic rituals that couples in real life Wife Led Marriages practice.
Worship Her: The daily vows that "Bow and Vow" says to his wife while kneeling before her each morning state everything that I feel and want to do each day for my wife. I will copy it down and try to memorize it this week to say to my goddess wife each day. It states what our WLM is about, and what I expect to do for her each day. I wouldn't change my worship for my wife for anything. The general male population of the world, if they read this vow, would laugh and think of us as fools. But we are the happiest men serving our wonderful wives. No domestic violence, no quarreling, just loving relationships, great respect for our wives and all women, and we have the happiest wives. All we want to do is please them in every way. What a great life we have! And they!
Anonymous: Yes, we are the happiest men serving our wives as it should be, unfortunately we are a minority. My friends take notice when I do wait on my wife at a party, refill her drink without being told, etc. They say so others can hear that I'm trying to make points with her because I want to get in her pants. If they only really knew that I'm not even allowed to beg or ask. Or that the following morning I will serve her coffee, clean the house, massage her (sometimes to her having an orgasm if that's what she wishes) and then take her shopping. No football on Sunday, just doing things with my wife instead. I wouldn't trade my life with theirs. We are the ones who are doing it right,

they are doing it wrong!

SK1111: I would love to have a ritual to kneel at my wife's feet and vow to serve her faithfully on a regular basis. She's running the show but still uncomfortable with acts of overt submission, but she does enjoy the massages, pedicures, etc., so I'm sure with time the Worship part will be enjoyed too.

Hopefully we will reach the day where I can serve her as my queen and she understands and accepts that she more than deserves all of it.

Worship Her: Even my wife who has dominated me for the last 8 years is also uncomfortable with me kneeling before her on a daily basis. She says it makes me look wimpy and she doesn't like it. So keep serving your wife, give her massages, and take her shopping and stay with her to help pick things out. She'll love that better.... Good luck to you, but I feel you already have it.

Anonymous: My wife and I have a FLM and having been doing it for about 5 years. We are both 54 years young and it has increased the romantic aspect of our marriage tenfold compared to others at our age. I do everything possible for her all of the housework after I come home from work. We lay in bed before going to sleep and we rub and caress each other, so much so that she usually ends up telling me to go down on her.

Runpb: Thanks for all the nice comments. I'm Mr. Remond's new email friend and I'm happy that others have enjoyed a glimpse into our beautiful marriage.

Steeredby: Since reading this I have knelt at her feet each morning before leaving for work. She kisses my forehead and I tell her I love her.

Mark: It has been inspiring and gratifying to read all your comments. The real credit, of course, goes to runpb for his beautifully crafted daily devotions.

3

GONNA TAKE AN
INCREMENTAL JOURNEY

Keep on Taking Those Baby Steps (6.12.08)

"Is there a point of no return when one truly embraces this way of life?"—"Ms. Kathleen," writing in Elise Sutton's *Predominant* e-magazine, February 2005 issue

A provocative question, especially for guys whose submissive yearnings are offset by their reservations and fears. Just how far down the FLR road dare they go before it's too late to turn around and scramble back to "the way things were"?

The journey, of course, starts with the first step. Most FLRs, I venture to say, were not inaugurated at one swell foop, but tentatively and incrementally. Whether the first steps are taken hand in hand, by mutual consent, or via stealth submission initiated by the husband, they're usually baby steps.

It's a good way to proceed, allowing both partners to adjust (consciously or subconsciously) to altered roles and power dynamics within the relationship. With a baby step, one foot can remain safely anchored in the comfort zone.

Emily and Ken Addison, co-creators of the *Around Her Finger* books and website and blog, recommend couples explore the lifestyle with a two-week "Boot Camp."

"During those two weeks," Emily advises an interested wife, "introduce him to loving female authority as described in the Boot Camp section of the book."

But, in order to achieve a full-fledged FLR, don't you need to stop "pussyfooting" around at some point and take some bold steps?

Yes, says Emily. "At the end of those two weeks, have an open and candid discussion about wife-led marriages and male submission. He will never want to go back to shared authority again."

Ultimately, the Addisons maintain, stealth submission is not sustainable. You need to take a Big Bold Step. Wife and husband need to affirm to each other that they are formally entering an FLR, not by tacit consent, but by mutual agreement. Most critically, the wife needs to assert her authority over her husband and her new status as head of the household, and the husband needs to acknowledge and accept this, going forward.

But why aren't baby steps enough, if you take enough of them? Well, according to a Pre-Socratic philosopher, Zeno of Elea, in a famous paradox, such incrementalism can never reach a goal:

"You cannot traverse an infinite number of points in a finite time. You must traverse the half of any given distance before you traverse the whole, and the half of that again before you can traverse it. This goes on *ad infinitum*, so that there are an infinite number of points in any given space, and you cannot touch an infinite number one by one in a finite time."

But let me disagree with the contemporary Addisons and ancient Zeno. The "half-the-distance" paradox holds true only in a theoretical universe. In fact, my college Greek Philosophy lecturer, who first told us about it, proceeded immediately to debunk it with a practical example:

Imagine the boys on one side of the class and girls on the other, and then imagine each side moving toward the other by traversing half the distance between them in a series of steps. Even though, in theory, they could never actually close the distance, as the lecturer explained, "after a relatively few steps the boys and girls would be close enough for all practical purposes."

Some very dramatic milestones, in other words, can be reached one step at a time. In the words of a famous haiku*:

O snail
Climb Mount Fuji,
But slowly, slowly!

(*by Kobayashi Issa, as translated by R.H. Blyth, quoted in J. D. Salinger's 1961 novel, *Franny and Zooey*.)

This isn't theory, because the baby-step method is exactly how I've proceeded in my own marriage. Often with a backward baby step for every two forward. In this halting fashion, my wife and I have covered a considerable distance. She is now in charge of almost every aspect of the marriage, our family life, my daily existence.

And we never, ever sat down and had that Talk. In fact, years ago whenever I would broach such a discussion, it almost always backfired. I stopped doing so.

I will acknowledge that sometimes the next baby step will turn out to have been a Big Step. Suddenly the climbing snail, inching upward, looks over his slimy shoulder and sees that it's a long, long way down... and then looks up and realizes he is dramatically closer to the summit.

I remember taking one of those next steps that suddenly loomed large and thinking, with a thrill, "This may be a point of no return on the road to wifedom."

Exactly what that step was is a topic for another post. But wanting to chroncle the milestone, I posted the following on a now-defunct female-led relationships board: "Finally, after more than a decade of on-again, off-again wife-worship, with incremental gains and losses, I realized we had turned the corner."

All those little steps had become a bold step. I and she and we were finally and actually committed to this lifestyle. Was I alarmed?

Maybe a wee bit. Like this husband, who wrote to Elise Sutton: "Dear Miss Sutton, I am coming to the realization that I am approaching a point of no return and each step, including reading your book, is taking me there."

Her advice: Fear not, but rejoice. "Do not fear submitting to a woman out of a fear of losing your male ego. Humility is a good thing for only a man who is humbled can than be edified to the place where he is fit for his Queen."

It's like an engagement. At some point, you need to call it off or march down the aisle. Commit to a wife-led marriage.

A wife-worshipping husband emailed me his realization when he saw where his own baby steps were leading:

"It really brought it home to me just how pleased and proud i was to be so completely controlled by the Woman who was irrevocably becoming my Mistress, how i/we had already gone beyond a point of no return, and how (deep down) i had always yearned for this ever since we met... It really made me feel in touch with my natural self, and even more accepting of who and what i am."

Maniac vs. Dilettante (7.1.08)

I've posted about taking "Baby Steps" and incremental wife worship, inching along, ever so slowly, the way the snail climbs Mt. Fuji.

Because, unless the idea for entering into a Female-Led Relationship originates with our wives, we husbands don't want to spook the objects of our adoration.

But, truth be told, Wife Worship is a form of psychological

mania, not a dilettantish pursuit or hobby. The idea, after all, is not simply to like and respect your wife, but to fall crazy nuts in love with her all over again—maybe even more truly, madly, deeply than the first time around.

To become obsessed by her... while—and this is the trick—contriving to appear pretty much sane and semi-normal in the process.

Walking the Walk (1.19.09)

When I began writing and publishing online the first chapters of *Worshipping Your Wife* more than eight years ago, I was mainly writing for the benefit of husbands, along with guys in committed relationships.

The idea was to offer these guys both a persuasive rationale and a step-by-step program for "Turning Marriage Back Into Passionate Courtship." I came up with six steps:

The husband needs to:

1. Realize that "the thrill is gone" and that he wants to get it back.

2. Save his sex energies for his wife.

3. Make *her* his fantasy.

4. Court her every day, attempt to win her anew.

5. Pamper her and pitch in around the house.

6. Dare to be known by her.

This was the progression that I myself had followed—or was in the process of following. In support of my six steps, I cited 'Net and newsgroup testimony posted pseudonymously over the years by worshipful husbands and worshipped wives, all of whom were busily practicing what I was still mainly theorizing about.

Happily, my own experience in the years since has confirmed

what I wrote in 2000, namely that "The transformations described in *Worshipping Your Wife* are real, the ideas workable..."

Does the program always work? Of course not. Sometimes it never even gets off the ground. Husbands who suddenly and enthusiastically spring this revolutionary notion all at once on an unsuspecting wife, whether in their own words or by handing her a book (like mine!), are likely to be met with healthy skepticism, maybe outright rejection. Where did all this weirdness come from?

Husbands who opt, on the other hand, for the cautious and incremental path to wife worship, a process often called "stealth submission," may encounter other obstacles. A few weeks of overzealous dishwashing and gift-giving may leave the wife in utter puzzlement. What's gotten into my Oswald?

Emily and Ken Addison describe this impasse clearly in their *Around Her Finger* books and on their blog:

"Women are very often confused by this approach. They ask their husbands what is behind the change in behavior, but their husbands have not yet mustered the courage to articulate their honest feelings... It is not enough for most [husbands] to simply undertake to serve and pamper their wives. There must be some explicit acknowledgement on the part of the woman [of her leadership in the marriage] or else the man is left unfulfilled."

For many guys, alas, it doesn't take much discouragement to get them to abandon the whole wife-worship campaign, stealthy or otherwise. The novelty and initial euphoria of doing housework wear off fast, and the wife's skepticism is thereby validated. Ditto for the husband whose wife hands back the FLR printout or book or impassioned confession with a firm No-Sale expression. He is likely to give up and go back to not worshipping her, unhappily ever after.

These husbands may ask themselves, Was it all imaginary? Was I just pretending to be this ultra-romantic guy who wanted to suddenly treat my wife like a queen?

Like this guy who asks: "What if I convince my wife to go

for this new arrangement where she's the queen of everything, and then I change my mind? What if serving her all the time was just a big, stupid fantasy after all?"

The answer, I guess, is that if you give up, it was never meant to be. You weren't sincere, it *was* just a fantasy, and you never really wanted it that bad. Whatever. And don't blame your wife for seeing through it, for not embracing a wild idea that you yourself were not committed to.

A husband in this quandary wrote for advice to Katherine West, who blogs occasionally at "Loving Female Authority." Her answer was forcefully to the point: "In a recent comment to one of my posts 'Quiet Guy' complains that his wife refuses to believe that he'll start doing more housework. Well, Quiet Guy, prove it to her. Get up at 4:00 a.m. and have it done before she's out of bed, if that's what it takes. [This] is very serious business. It is not a game. Until she's received her 52nd foot rub from you, until you've made some token confession of your [total devotion], until you have made every effort to prove to her that you are there to serve her, then don't give up."

Another wife gives a similar response in a letter to the Addisons' "Around Her Finger" blog: "About four years ago [my husband] tried to communicate his feelings to me [about wanting a wife-led marriage]. He did a good job. But what he said and how day to day life was lived were two different things... It wasn't until my husband actually started walking the walk and not just talking the talk did I take [him] seriously. He started doing the housework, running the errands, all the things I had done for the past 24 years."

You can't just close the deal, in other words, on the basis of a feverish sales pitch accompanied by sales pamphlets full of glowing testimonials from happy wife-worship customers. Talk is cheap, as Liza Dolittle sings to Freddy Eysford Hill in *My Fair Lady*: "Show me now!"

Which is exactly what this devoted husband did in a successful "stealth" campaign that lasted many years:

"To convince my wife that I truly wanted to worship and

serve her as my queen took years of dedication to housework, child-rearing and pampering without any thought of reward. I did the chores cheerfully and enthusiastically. Yet, each time I failed and became lazy, I felt that I took several steps backward for both of us. I was moving from one equilibrium to another in terms of our relationship, and I needed to be perfect, not anything in between, not just sometimes. Ultimately I convinced her that this was my life, that I was fulfilled in that role and didn't want anything other than to worship and serve her."

"I decided I could not create a female-led relationship," writes another husband. "I wonder if any man can. What I did decide is that I could be in a male-following relationship... So I settled in to serving my wife and doing my best to obey her will whether she asserted it dominantly or not. I truly had no expectation that she would change her behavior. The funny thing was that, almost immediately after I made this change, my wife changed as well [becoming comfortable in a leading role]."

A last word on the topic from another husband: "It took many years for us to learn how to get along and build a new relationship... Like the Nike add says, 'Just Do It.'"

Comments:
Whatevershesays: Male following is the key, but it's so damn hard. And there is a balance between male following and the need for the wife to actively acknowledge that she is in charge. And yes, this active acknowledgment must involve some type of sexuality.

Mark: I agree that at some point the husband needs some kind of active acknowledgment from the worshiped wife. But if she goes along and accepts the adoration, the service and the surrender of decision-making and takes charge more and more... well, you've at least got the game without the name. I know of a couple marriages, including my own, where that is the case, and the other hubby and I are not frustrated but rather grateful for what we have, and are both disinclined to push any further, in order to comply with anyone else's pre-requisites to be adjudged a Compleat FLR. On the contrary, when I start listing all that has been achieved and acknowledged, I am overwhelmed with gratitude... and yes, sex is involved, too.

But I suspect we are probably in agreement, beneath all my verbiage.

At All Times: I suspect that most relationships where the wife knows of her husband's submissive tendencies will over time develop in such a way that the wife will take advantage of the fact that she knows that she is in a strong position, and in this way will acknowledge or demonstrate her position of power more freely and openly. The husband's role is surely to remain attentive and prove his submission by accepting her rule. It may not be the mind-blowing, or most exciting sexual fantasy life that you ever imagined, but at least you will be fulfilling the most basic of wife-led marriage principles that your wife has control.

SK1111: I too think it's important to communicate your submission, then it's follow your wife's lead. She will develop things as she see fit and becomes comfortable with her position and what it grants her... She will move at her pace and with luck you'll get the relationship of your dreams over time, but don't rush it, she needs to de-program that conventional thinking we all got fed while growing up. If she does you will be blessed.

Falling in Love Again (10.9.09)

"Perpetual Courtship," a chapter title in Worshipping *Your Wife*, could easily serve as the book's title. "PC" is pretty much what "wife worship" is all about. As Fumika Misato says on her "Real Women Don't..." website, "This is a marriage in which your husband courts you until death do you part."

But when I say "perpetual courtship," does that mean the suitor's goal is never to be reached? Is the lady to be endlessly wooed, never won?

My answer is that yes, there *is* a goal, and yes, she is to be won—over and over again. Why not slay a dragon-a-day to prove your mettle?

But there's another way to look at this ongoing courtship, especially for husbands whose wives are initially unreceptive to the notion of a female-led relationship, as presented. It's "stealth courtship," often termed "stealth submission."

Without a word to his wife, the stealthy husband-suitor begins incrementally and unilaterally taking on household chores, giving her more respect, paying attention to her whims and wishes, buying her special gifts, complimenting her, etc.

He begins practicing, in other words, many of the behaviors I codified into my book's "Six Steps for Turning Marriage Back Into Passionate Courtship."

The problem with such courtship, or "stealth submission," according to Ken and Emily Addison of the *Around Her Finger* book and blog, is that it's not sustainable. The Addisons seem adamant that wife and husband need to affirm to each other at the outset that they are formally entering an FLR, not by tacit consent, but by mutual agreement. Most critically, the wife needs to assert her authority over her husband and her new status as head of the household, and the husband needs to acknowledge and accept this, going forward.

That's a bit like saying courtship can't be sustained if the girl doesn't say "yes" to the first proposal. How many marriages would never have come to pass if the guy gave up at the first "no"? Old-time Fuller Brush salesmen were trained to get past three, four, five, even six "no's" at the front door and still close a sale. Can a suitor do less to make the sale of his life?

So, yes, the recommendation here is for a second courtship of one's wife or girlfriend, not only with the idea that she must be won anew, but that she must be assiduously courted by a new suitor, a new "you." With the idea that, ultimately, she will fall in love with that new you.

A little weird, yes, and like the Addisons say, hard to keep up day after day, perhaps with little encouragement. But if it is sustained, stealth courtship can prevail. A wife, initially skeptical ("Is this guy really my Fred, or some Alien Replicant?"), can learn to love being treated like a queen, can fall in love all over again with a different version of her husband. She can and likely will gradually grow comfortable with having more and more power in the relationship, where her wishes are supreme, her decisions are final and domestic tranquility prevails.

In romantic obsession, the would-be wife worshipper usually outstrips any "vanilla" suitor, including himself the first time around. As Misato informs interested wives, "You will find that this new relationship goes far beyond the courtship that you experienced when dating."

Enough theory. Here it is in practice, an example of a wife falling in love with a new version of her husband, as told from the woman's point of view. It appeared in the blog "Giving Up Control—Female Led Life," which is cowritten by wife (Ladyof7, "Lo7") and husband (kept by 7, "Kb7"). Here is Ladyof7's version:

"I have come to 'prefer' the submissive edge to Kb7 over the vanilla Kb7. Who wouldn't love a husband who has you sitting upon a pedestal catering to your every whim, and agreeing with everything you say without a question? Don't get me wrong, the vanilla Kb7 is who I fell in love with to begin with, but someone better has come along so to speak. I have fallen out of love with the vanilla Kb7 and fell very much in love with the new life I have with Kb7... I am having fun with the lifestyle I have become committed to, and I wonder if we can continue on with this forever."

This, by the way, is the courtship path that I have also pursued, albeit incrementally and circuitously and with far less consistency than I should. But, as I think I have mentioned before, when I look at the way we are now, my wonderful wife and I, and the way we were when this all started, it is clear that all those hesitant baby steps have led me deep and irrevocably into the Queendom of Matriarchy.

Comments:

I Worship Her: About 4 years ago, I began a stealth WLR with my wife of 26 years. I did everything for her, sometimes overdid it to her annoyance, and finally seemed to get just the right amount of submissiveness she was comfortable with... So be patient, show your wives how wonderful it can be, don't overdo it at first. It will take many months. But she will love it and never want to go back. My wife is now quite dominant in our WLR, practices strict orgasm control on me. I do all of the housework while she sits and watches me, reads or watches tv. I prepare many of our meals, massage her feet and wherever else she desires, never argue with her because I will always accept her point of view, take her shopping at my request and stay with her to pick out clothes or to get different sizes. No husbands' chair, she puts me to work. We are happier the last few years than we could ever imagine, closer than ever before, and have the best relationship a husband and wife could hope for. So take your time and you too will develop a great WLR!

He Worships Me: I told my husband to send in his story (above) of how we began our WLR. I never knew what was behind his submissive change, and yes, at times he tried to do too much for me that I did get very annoyed at him. I found it unusual that when I got very annoyed or angry, he would hear me out, say he was sorry and drop it. Nothing like what he would have done in the past. Now when I get in a bad mood, instead of him annoying me or even ignoring me, he talks to me and will always find something to do to change my attitude. I guess because I am more dominant now and he is submissive, I really don't get into bad moods. He is always there to please me. And when you come home and see your husband dusting or cleaning the floors or preparing drinks and dinner, there are no bad moods. Ours is based on love, respect and trust. What better qualities could you have in a WLR?

Mark: What a coup to get husband-and-wife postings. These comments should certainly encourage husbands that a wife-governed marriage can be in their future, either by confessing all or by proceeding in stealthy baby steps to begin serving her now. In fact, confessing all really should be proceeded by weeks of conscientious solicitude on behalf of one's wife.

Anonymous: I can't imagine how hard it must be to confess something so personal, even to a spouse. My boyfriend was terrified. This wasn't the sort of thing, in his mind, that macho jock types were supposed to want. He was afraid that I would lose respect for him, be turned off, or any number of crazy things. However, I can't imagine any woman not going for FLR once it's been properly explained. Sure, it runs sort of contrary to societal norms, but it offers so many benefits (better sex, more attentiveness, and communication) that all the so-called pitfalls hardly feel like pitfalls at all.

Maybe it's a generational thing. My boyfriend introduced me to this dynamic a little under a year ago, but we've only recently finished college. I can see how a liberal-ish college girl might have an easier time adjusting to FLR than, say, a conservative, 45-year-old who feels that female leadership is immoral. Hopefully, that will change in the future. Having tasted the forbidden fruit, so to speak, I can't see myself ever going back. I'm sure that many women of all backgrounds would feel the same way if they just opened their minds and gave it a chance.

4

SURRENDERING THE SWORD

Caught in the Courtship Loop, Part 1 (4.25.09)

The animating idea of my book, *Worshipping Your Wife*, is that the magic of first love does not have to wear off. And, darn it, if it does, it can be recaptured and perpetuated. Yea, verily, a husband and wife can reinfect one another with honeymoon fever even unto the happy-ever-aftering of storybooks and Harlequin romances, until death do them part.

I lifted this hopeful concept, with I hope appropriate acknowledgment, from the website of Fumika Misato ("Real Women Don't Do Housework"). A great many variants of this life-changing idea can be found also on FLR websites, repeated in testimonials posted online in newsgroups, bulletin boards and in many emails to me by worshipful husbands and their worshipped wives.

"Perpetual Courtship," I call it in the book. Think of *Ground Hog Day* meets *50 First Dates*. The husband wakes up each morning with an overwhelming urge (and need) to resume his hormone-fueled courtship of his wife, to win her all over again, as if for the first time.

I prescribe various kinds of courtship behaviors that ardent hubbies can keep practicing, in an endless romantic loop.

But, you may ask, can't this get a little déjà-vuish? Yes, it can. And, speaking guy-wise, it is especially hard to wake up après sex and launch into a full-court, courtship press. "You mean, we gotta win her all over again?" the hormones are apt to complain. "We're not exactly in the mood right now."

This is why Lady Misato counsels wives to master the art of keeping their husbands sexually "on edge":

"As a general rule," she writes, "you will elicit the best behavior from your husband if you keep him on the edge between frustration and satisfaction... A husband who is sexually satisfied will have no energy to attend to your needs."

The same prescription is given by Emily and Ken Addison of the *Around Her Finger* website, books and CDs. "My husband is the perfect man until after he has an orgasm," a woman writes to Emily, "then he rolls over like the ape that he was before we discovered your site. Is this normal?"

Keep him on edge, Emily replies. "It is no great secret that after sex men become very sleepy and disinterested in affection and communication... [but] I promise that any man that is denied an orgasm will have no desire whatsoever to get quickly off to sleep after being intimate with his wife... He will dote on his wife, playing with her hair, rubbing her back, and kissing her neck and shoulders. He will behave as if he is just getting to know her. It will be as if the old flames have been rekindled."

It's the "uncertainty principle" at work, according to one Internet couples counselor calling herself "Dr. Ann" (quoted in chapter 4 of my book, "A Playful Step Beyond"): "When my female clients add the uncertainty principle of arousal and denial to their marriage, a woman can bring her husband back to the days when they were first dating."

"Forcing a buildup of semen in men should be the goal of all females," another controlling wife says simply. "Your man's behavior toward you will change dramatically for the better as his semen levels increase. You should always deny your man an orgasm prior to events that might require his maximum male energy and aggressiveness." This, by the way, is pretty much the standard advice boxers are given by their trainers on the runup to a big fight. To help enforce it, fighters often are sent to hideaway training camps, far from feminine temptation.

But does perpetual courtship require perpetual denial? The answer, thank God, is no, and I have it on the authority of those two leading lights of the Loving Female Authority movement, Fumika Misato and Elise Sutton.

Let's start with Misato: "You absolutely do not want to frustrate your husband for too long. If your husband becomes overly frustrated, he will be tempted to seek relief outside the marriage. On the other hand, you do not want to overly satisfy him either. A husband who is sexually satisfied will have no energy to attend to your needs. Finding the right balance of sexual desire is tricky."

Which, not surprisingly, is pretty much chapter and verse the advice from Elise Sutton: "You have to find the balance that works for your relationship. You have discovered that your husband is balanced when you give him an orgasm every two to three weeks. That is great. With my husband, once a month works. Why don't I deny him longer? Because through experimentation I have discovered that it becomes counterproductive to go longer than that. Some women allow their man an orgasm once a week. Some women can deny their husbands for months at a time... It all boils down to what works with your man."

The process works, even when the husband knows he is being manipulated: "My lovely wife has it pretty well figured out that much more than a week begins to be counterproductive," a happy husband writes. "She also understands that, as Lady Misato advises, she must continually keep me 'on the edge.'"

Some guys, as Elise Sutton indicated, are made to endure longer periods of enforced abstinence: "I have been denied an orgasm for four weeks and it has caused me to be in touch and in sync with her moods, wants and demands. So far, I regularly do the dishes, the laundry, get the kids ready and out to school, and basically all of the kitchen chores. She doesn't have to hound me to do any of it."

This husband exhibits other classic symptoms of the courting male: "I find myself going nuts to attract her attention. Over the summer I lost a lot of weight and am about 14 lb. short of my ideal. I almost look as fit as when we met."

"I feel more focused, alive, vital, and sexual when I am denied regular orgasms by my wonderful wife. When I come too often, I become torpid, disaffected, and disinterested in her. Far better to be kept tantalizingly on edge."

Another teased-and-denied husband echoes this: "I do not perform for my wife as well when I come too often. I have been living this lifestyle long enough to know that denial by our dominant wives for us is one of the most effective things."

"My wife has been keeping me on edge constantly, and although I never would have predicted it, I love it. She has me waiting on her hand and foot, doting on her constantly, and sexually it has become all about her, as it should be."

So, is the ultimate happy-ever-after marriage an endless replay of courtship? Perhaps surprisingly, my answer is no. But I'll save the explanation for the next post.

Comments:

Anonymous: I encourage [my husband] to read every word of each post. (Well, I actually demand he do it.) I have a motto that we live by in our house, "a horny husband is a good husband." I make him wait a minimum of one month, longer if he has displeased me in any way during that time frame. He will be punished by waiting an additional week or weeks. That rarely happens, though, because he is totally in favor of wife worship and strives to please me in every way possible with no expectations for himself. He is very well trained, and we have a very loving relationship, one that all of my friends are in envy of. Our lives have never been better since we began practicing wife worship about four years ago, and we have been married for 36 years. We are both in our late 50's, the children are married or on their own. So he and I are alone in our house which makes wife worship very easy to do 24/7.

Mark: I'm sure I'm not alone among the male readers here in envying your husband. And, of course, I was especially tickled to know that you are both reading and enjoying the blog posts.

Caught in the Courtship Loop, Part 2 (5.27.09)

Part 1 of this posting ended with a question: Is the ultimate happy-ever-after marriage an endless replay of courtship? An endless blissful loop, in other words, a la *Groundhog Day*?

That's certainly the answer implied in my book's final chapter, "Happy-Ever-Aftering Takes Work": "Fumika Misato seems quite confident about the prospects for happy-ever-aftering. She tells wives: 'This is a marriage in which your husband courts you till death does you part.'"

But that can't be right—an endless loop, or freeze frame. Things don't remain status quo for that long. They change, evolve, devolve, whatever. Here, just for the heck of it, are a few metaphysical quotes to that effect:

"Everything flows and nothing remains the same."—Heraclitus

"Nothing can develop by staying on one level...Nothing in the world stays in the same place, or remains what it was; everything moves, everything is going somewhere, is changing, and inevitably either develops or weakens."—G. I. Gurdjieff

"You define a thing by the direction it is going."—James Paige

The real answer is that I don't know the answer—what the ultimate condition of a courtship marriage is or can be. But my inclination is that happy-every-aftering is not an endless ground hog day of courtship, even though those elements are perpetuated. My sense is that the courtship marriage, like any other relationship, needs to grow and deepen or it will decline.

So, if it is to grow, in what way? I have written that passion need not ebb. And I believe it. But if you measure passion by testosterone levels, then I grant you that ebbing is pretty inevitable, given the sales trendlines for Viagra and Cialis *et al.,* (with similar products more quietly marketed for women).

"We used to do it all night, and now it takes us all night to do it," goes the old joke, and it's true enough. But there is a silver lining to this graying of passion. As Elise Sutton writes: "As a man ages, his sex drive diminishes as he loses testosterone. But as his physical sex drive may diminish, his mental desire for sex does not... You can now gain mental, emotional, social and spiritual fulfillment via serving a woman. That may mean doing chores for her, obeying her authority, pampering her and also sexually serving her."

Wife worship, in other words, is not dependent on testosterone levels. Even with a diminished sexual drive, a romantically inflamed imagination, according to Ms. Sutton, can keep a man "devoted and committed to the woman in his life." "And that," she adds, "empowers the woman."

So, in a wife worship marriage, an aging husband can feel as giddy and adoring as a honeymooner, even if the manifestations of that desire are less obvious.

Now I am old enough to have experienced this alternation of passion, so I can tell you that Elise Sutton is right. And I'm not alone in my testimony:

"After all these years of worshipping my wife," a husband confides in a wife-led marriage forum, "she has gradually been elevated to almost Goddess status in my eyes. I find that our sexuality is more on a mental sphere than a physical one and I worship her in spirit and in the flesh."

On a more mundane level, there is also a feeling of being "comfortable." My love for my wife, as in any happy and long-enduring marriage, tends to become an ever-present thing. And yet, it does seem to progress. I experience a slow, incremental drawing-closer to her, a devotional pull that reminds me of the "tractor beam" that pulled Luke Skywalker and his Millenium Falcon friends inexorably toward the Death Star. Except, of course, you must picture, in place of that dark nexus of evil, a radiant and glorious and good She-goddess, into whose intoxicating orbit you are being drawn.

It's like penetrative sex, don't you know? She is the divine ovum, and you are the frenetic, lost spermatozoon, desperately seeking... well, let's call it amalgamation. Sex as daily metaphor, with you becoming more and more a part of your wife, living within her orbit and aura.

As this intimacy grows and abides into later life, of course, a wife worship marriage is going to be preoccupied with the practicalities of any aging couple—launching the kids, financing college, securing retirement, paying off the mortgage, arranging adequate health care, staying well and busy, etc. But even these exigencies can be tinted with an enduring honeymoon glow.

Comments:

Bob: Thank you for talking about romance and love in a blog about female supremacy. This does not happen on most blogs about matriarchy. I also appreciate you focusing on the everyday aspect of life, like housework and girl's night out and simple interactions between husband and wife.

Mark: I do try to concentrate on the romantic aspects of what Lady Misato first termed "wife worship," not where this lifestyle can veer far away from the mainstream.

Whatevershesays: Nicely done. Courtship doesn't have to end. Don't know what I would do if it did.

Art: Here's to growing older and closer!

Rex: Here's to growing older and closer to the center of her gravity.

Big 'O' Overrated? (3.5.09)

The "Big O" for a lot of guys of a certain age instantly conjures up the Cincinnati Royals' basketball legend Oscar Robertson, once widely considered the game's greatest all-around player. That was, of course, way before the advent of Dr. J, Bird, Magic, MJ, Kobie, Le Bron, et al.

Was Oscar overrated? No way. He really *was* that great.

But that's not the "Big O" under re-evaluation here. I'm talking about the male orgasm. Not knocking it, heaven forefend, but matched up against the female orgasm, the "Bigger O," does ours really deserve top spot on the awards podium?

Let's not delve too deeply into point-by-point matchups—frequency, degree of intensity, duration, etc. You can look all that up. The consensus seems pretty clear: Guys come in a distant second on the Bliss-O-Meter in all these comparisons, bigtime.

Unless—and here's my point—we opt to go with the female flow... hang on for dear life... and surf along on the breaking crest of our partner's orgasmic tsunami (sorry, I'm getting really carried away)... till it finally subsides... way the hell up the beach.

In other words, make her ecstasy *your* ecstasy. To the extent that we even forget (at least temporarily) about our own. To the extent that we are truly fulfilled by being a part of her powerful, all-encompassing completion.

I don't want to give myself too much credit here, but I've always pretty much felt this way, from the moment I vicariously experienced my first female orgasm. It was a revelation, a redefinition of "peak experience." The notion that I had been involved in, or a facilitator of, anything so rapturousy cataclysmic made me feel like a superhero.

Still does. That's what I daydream about when I think of sex—*hers*, not mine.

And those early formative experiences came during an era when the ideal of ultimate hetero-sex was the simultaneous climax—after, of course, a long interlocking gallop. It acquired near-mythic status in popular culture, starting with Papa Hemingway (*For Whom the Bell Tolls*: "Come now, now, for there is no now but now. Yes, now. Now, please now....") and his legion of schlocky imitators, to all those erotic cinematic climax-montages dissolving into

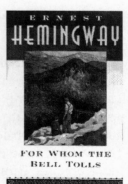

FOR WHOM THE
BELL TOLLS

72

the shared, post-coital cigarette.

Not knocking it again, but, like the *de rigueur* vaginal climax, this kind of seismic togetherness doesn't happen as often in real life as in books and movies.

These days sexual synchronicity is being replaced by another paradigm, which is neatly encapsulated in the title of one popular book, *She Comes First: The Thinking Man's Guide to Pleasuring a Woman* by Ian Kerner.

Wife-worshippers along with advocates of Wife-Led Marriages and Female-Led Relationships take this prescription a bit farther. Like, for instance, She comes first... and second... maybe even third.

And what about her partner in passion? He is admonished to be patient, be a good boy, and wait for her to give him the green light.

Is this a good thing? A lot of men say that it is. I joined that chorus myself in my book, especially Chapter 4, "A Playful Step Beyond": "...[it] extends and intensifies the husband's pleasure, saving him from a quick release followed by an even quicker loss of desire—climax and anti-climax."

"Save yourself for her direction," I quote a happy husband as advising another chap. "Your satisfaction will be intensified."

And here is complementary advice from a woman whose husband has now learned to worship her as his queen: "[The woman] should never feel that denying her male orgasm for long periods of time is overly cruel. In fact, rather than cruelty, long-term orgasm denial is a gift she provides her male. When the male achieves orgasm it is accompanied by a release of all sexual tension. As being in a state of sexual tension is so blissful, the male orgasm is always to one extent or another a disappointment."

This hubby definitely concurs: "People ask me how I can go so long without sex. They don't get that my wife and I are having sex pretty much 24/7, we just go a long time between orgasms. Making my Goddess have orgasms is one of the greatest feelings in the world for me. God, I love my life!"

And one final hurrah for the Female O: "I pleasured my queen this a.m. and without a word she just fell asleep when she was done. It makes me feel great to experience her orgasm, and then to see her relax that much and to know that I've contributed to it by not making demands on her for my pleasure."

Comments:
Anonymous: Thank you for this witness of the value of women's orgasms.
Mark: I'm happy to be among the cheering male multitude at the glories of the female orgasm.
Ms. Rayne: I agree with you. Sexual tension is delicious. I think the sensation makes men hyper aware.
Anonymous: The hornier the husband, the better the husband. I keep my husband very horny, for a month or more. Is he ever on good behavior! Yes, he does wear a chastity device for a little added protection—this was totally his idea. He is not allowed to ask out of it, complain about it, or ask for any release. These are my decisions.
PM: I have stopped using the term "orgasm" equally for both male and female sexual experience, as I do not think they can be equated that easily. Rather than an emotional love-based orgasm, [the male's] is strictly speaking merely an insemination reflex. It lasts for a much shorter time and is far less intense than our female climax, and for these qualitative reasons alone it does not deserve the same term. A glass of water and a vitamin pill are just not the same as a full candlelit dinner with violin accompaniment...

Even more important on a psychological relationship level, this male pleasure at ejaculation is also a much more selfish one. Is it not very often true that men after their "orgasm" are much less devoted to their wives and thus to their relationship commitments? That is really the most important reason to keep them chaste—in order to strengthen the couple relationship. Most women, on the other hand, feel confirmed in the love of their partner, their relationship and also much more loving to their partners after a good orgasm.

So in my view it is only this positive female orgasm that both partners should strive for in any sexual activity. To reinforce that fact, I think, both male and female partners should refer to it not as "her" or "my" orgasm but "our orgasm," as in: "Darling, how was our Orgasm?"

There are some nice parallels to people speaking of "our baby" even though it is mainly the woman who experiences pregnancy and the man contributed very little at the beginning. Still a baby is definitely a couple thing, like an orgasm, and not just "his sperm" and "her ovum." Both worked for it in their own special way, and they both equally share the enjoyment of it.

Please do not think that what I am saying here is that the male sexual climax is unimportant. First, it is vital for the reproduction of the species, as it is still the cheapest and most fun way to get pregnant. Also we should not underestimate the evolutionary need of the male for his pleasure. It initially provides much of the male's motivation for contributing to a relationship and is a vital part of making the chastity lifestyle work for you both.

[But] the selfish nature of the actual male sexual release as opposed to the loving behaviour exhibited by males just dreaming of it, is another reason why I think that when it comes to male sexual climax, the disappointing and somewhat destructive actual event is to be avoided as much as possible. The pleasurable and positive myth, on the other hand, is to be built up as much as possible by all means available (both physical and psychological teasing).

I do not think the male climax should ever be more than an occasional tip for very good behaviour, and men should never be able to take it for granted, let alone be misled into believing his climax to be anywhere near orgasmic or anywhere near as important in the couple relationship.

Mark: *You* should be writing a book or blog on the topic of female-led relationships. Please, PM, encore!

Changing Male Behavior, Part 1 (9.6.08)

"She'd gone and picked another guy with major hangups. According to her girlfriend, she had a thing for such reclamation projects. But weren't all men basically projects?"

I think there's some truth to that last statement, even if I wrote it myself (in an unpublished novel). Lord knows I was, and am, a project for my wife. I look back on our wedding and wonder, Did she know then how much remodeling it would take for her to properly domesticate me and make me fit for cohabitation? Did she have a plan, a blueprint, a timeline?

One of these days maybe I'll ask her.

And yet, sweet young things are often counseled against marrying a man with the expectation of changing him. This so-called truism was even codified as Rule No. 18 in *The Rules: Time-*

Tested Secrets for Capturing the Heart of Mr. Right, Ellen Fein and Sherrie Schneider's 1995 best-seller: "Don't Expect a Man to Change or Try to Change Him." The co-authors promise happy relationships and happy marriages to the readers who follow their 35 specific rules.

Apparently, the idea of changing male behavior is a kind of psychological heresy. But changing male behavior for a successful and lasting romantic relationship is not only doable, it's essential. (Notice, I'm *not* suggesting the feasibility or necessity of changing male nature, which is hard-wired; on the contrary, my prescriptions for changing male behavior are based on understanding and exploiting male nature.)

I codified a couple of essential behavioral changes as Steps 2 & 3 in *Worshipping Your Wife: Six Steps for Turning Marriage Back Into Passionate Courtship* (alas, not a best-seller, not yet anyway):

Step 2: Save His Sex Energies For His Wife.
Step 3: Make *Her* His Fantasy

These two steps can lead to big-time changes—gynormous changes—in terms of romantically and sexually binding the husband to his wife for the duration.

And they can be accomplished, either unilaterally, with conscious and unflagging effort by an ardent husband intent on putting the magic back in his marriage (the approach in my book). Or by a wife, consciously applying those same principles, with or without the husband's consent (the approach of Lady Misato on her website, "Real Women Don't Do Housework."

Thess may seem like exotic or radical notions, but are they really? It's hardly Headline News that men can be manipulated by women. Isn't that what women have been doing from Eden onward, lo these many millennia? Isn't that their job?

In Chapter One of my book I quote philosopher George Gilder to precisely that effect: "Women manipulate male sexual desire in order to teach men the long-term cycles of female sexuality and biology on which civilization is based."

I found elements of this idea, elaborated on with a personal slant, on a female supremacy message board years ago attributed to "Goddess M":

"As females we need to admit to ourselves that we all have a desire to change our male. We want him to more often exhibit behaviors which please us, and less frequently exhibit behaviors that are displeasing to us.

"[But] females are taught by society that it is not right to want to change the male, and that even if it were ethical, it can't be done anyway. The conclusion we are to draw is that if we try to change our male our efforts will fail and we will be deeply disappointed.

"This is a lie, a lie of course foisted upon females by our prevailing patriarchal society... As females, control of the male orgasm is our best opportunity to improve our male's behavior patterns and mold him more closely into the 'man of our dreams'... Through enforced chastity we can change the male with relative ease, and we should do so... His instincts will drive him to exhibiting pleasing behavior towards her, and will make it much more difficult for him to exhibit behaviors which she does not approve of."

The amazing thing is, men love to be manipulated in this way. On her website (now celebrating its first decade), Lady Misato has many testimonials to that effect. Let me excerpt just two:

"Dear Lady Misato, [My wife] has taken control outside of the bedroom, using sex to condition me to her will...My life has changed, perhaps forever. My wife is wonderful. I am amazed at her erotic power and her skill at wielding it... Your method is powerful and her implementation, flawless. I am hers to do with as she will, and she knows it. Do I like to admit that? Not one bit! Can I do anything otherwise? Not at all."

And a wife writes: "I just started trying your technique on my hubby and am amazed at how well it works! He has figured out exactly what I am doing, but, just as you said, he seems compelled to submit. It's wonderful!! Thank you!"

So what kind of changes are we talking about?

I'll give some examples in Part 2 of this posting.

Changing Male Behavior, Part 2 (9.11.08)

I promised (in Part 1 of this posting) to give some radical changes in male behavior that are eminently achievable through wife worship, whether that worship be initiated by ardent husband or demanding wife. So here, courtesy of Lady Misato's "Real Women Don't Do Housework," we go:

According to this wife, "I freely ask my husband to do things like clear the dishes, mop the floor, iron the clothes... I don't give it a second thought. My husband obeys without question always. A few days ago, I was pleased to have overheard his conversation with one of my lady friends after we had dinner at home. She asked if he always does all this work around the house (washing, clearing the dishes, etc.). He replied that he does and enjoys doing it. When she asked why? He said it was because I wanted him to and that it made me happy. And the look on my friend's face turned from amusement to genuine amazement."

A husband confesses: "I do most of the housework now. I don't consider this a chore but a pleasure. I owe her so much and love her so much that I enjoy doing everything I can. Her sensual hold on me is very real and while sometimes I have trouble distinguishing what is caused by my love for her and what is more guided by my sexual drive towards her, the end result is the same: I listen, respond, obey, and love every minute of it."

Some wives work these changes without benefit of my book, or Lady Misato's or any website, just by instinct, like the wife of Au876, a worshipful husband often quoted here:

"I am not real sure how our marriage evolved into Wife Worship. It started out with me as the king of my castle though I strived to make sure she had her say. [But] when I started doing more of 'my share' of the chores, I found she was very appreciative. She not only rewarded me, she began to encourage me. Today I not only do all the housework and cooking, I perform many personal chores for her and am always seeking more ways to please her. I truly worship her and have eyes for no other woman."

Au writes that, before this transformation, "I had the same shopping problems [as most guys]. Mostly shopping is just not a 'man' thing. We know what we want, go get it and get out. But that has changed now. I go with my wife (if invited—sometimes she likes to go alone). I carry the packages. The last time she went clothes shopping about two months ago, she got a bunch of clothes to try on. They only allowed two things in the dressing room at a time. I stood outside her dressing cubicle. She'd try on something, send me to get a different size or color, put it in the 'to buy' stack or back on the rack. Several times she sent me to get a certain color shoe to see how the dress went with them. Several other customers were struggling with trying on clothes without the help of their husbands. I found myself busting with pride to be so much help to my wife."

What technique did Mrs. Au876 utilize? Did it involve controlling his sexual release? You darned betcha:

"She controls my sex life. After less than a week of no sex she can touch me and I am an instant total erection. After about ten days she can look at me and have me trembling with desire, a forbidden desire I know she controls. I throb for her, my face, my whole body ache for her. But I am denied release simply because she controls me. How do I stand it? I worship and adore her all the more as I focus on pleasing her. It is my duty. And I am no longer bored with it. I get excited washing dishes, washing her underwear, rubbing her feet or running her errands. Somebody recently wrote me in this forum saying my wife had me by the balls. I guess she does. But I know what she expects of me and I do it, or at least I try too."

Pretty dramatic changes—not in male nature, but male behavior. I'm not in Au876's league, nor does my wife desire to emulate Au's wife. But if I were to jot down all the positive changes in attitude and performance that have been worked in recent years, it would make an impressive list.

And I'm not through yet, nor is she. Work on the unfinished husband project continues.

Comments:

Jboy: An important topic. Changing male behavior is exactly what FLR is all about. It is a Woman's right to change her hubby for the sake of her own happiness and for his. A bride becomes an artist who molds her hubby into a loving, obedient and well domesticated boy who devotes himself to his Wife. He will find true happiness and fulfillment in being molded by her skilled hands and pride in becoming her prized possession.

Mr. Manhers: As She is his fantasy, it's only sensible for him to do as she wishes to fulfill hers.

Mark: In fact, it is difficult for me to conjure up the person I was when we married, so much has she altered who I am, without really trying. I mean, the changes have simply been worked on me, I think, through the force of her own personality and superior judgment and resolve. I do remember quarreling with her, early on, and taking stands on this and that, invariably caving and apologizing and doing exactly as she had originally proposed.

5

IN HER MAJESTY'S
SACRED SERVICE

In Her World (4.9.09)

"[My wife] has arrived home and my heart is fluttering with excitement! I hurry to do her bidding. I do not feel complete until she is home. I'm near the center of the feminine mystery, an intimate part of the life of a beautiful woman. So close to her, caring only for her comfort and happiness." ("Near the Center of the Feminine Mystery," included in Chapter 17 of this book.)

"Harry was transferred to the feminine department, where his life was little short of heavenly... He took a pride in servility to a beautiful woman; received Lady Vandeleur's commands as so many marks of favour... to pass one's days with a delicate woman, and principally occupied about trimmings, was to inhabit an enchanted isle among the storms of life." (From "Story of the Bandbox" by Robert Louis Stevenson, posted back on January 5, 2007 under "RLS and the Enchanted Isle," see Chapter 17 of this book.)

Not very macho, the giddy husband with his heart a-flutter on his wife' s return home, or Harry, currying the favor of beautiful Lady Vandeleur.

Contrast these lightweights with a real macho husband. He

comes back from a long sales trip to find his wife has redecorated their all-American bedroom in a Continental style, inspired by interior design magazines. He throws a fit, demands she remove every last ruffle and pastel what-have-you and put everything back the way it was. He's not going to sleep in some "goddamned Parisian bordello."

Does that sounds like a sitcom episode of, say, "Married With Children"? Waiting for the chauvinist jerk to get his comeuppance? But sixty years or so ago, when this story reportedly took place, autocratic husbands could get away with stuff like that. These days, the guy could call himself lucky if his wife set aside one room as "an estrogen-free zone"—the den, say, complete with Laz-E-Boy and "Dogs Playing Poker" wall art.

While the rest of the house is the Lair of the She-Creature. Which is just fine with wife-worshipping husbands. We enjoy inhabiting "Lady Vandeleur's enchanted island."

Maybe we're secure enough in our masculinity that we don't need to have it constantly reinforced and reflected back at us. We're not threatened by chintz and organza, bedskirts and dust ruffles. These are clues that we are drawing "near the center of the feminine mystery, an intimate part of the life of a beautiful woman."

Now some quotes, staring with this one from my book, Chapter 5. "Pampering and Pitching In":

"Men are fascinated with a woman's body. They want to be a part of it and to understand it. Often sex is a type of adoration and respect for woman... He longs for her to teach him about the great mystery of woman."

"She wrapped Her Arm around me and put my head on Her Chest. i was feeling much better now. In the silence, i could sense the relaxation spreading through my body. my life was once again back in Her capable Hands! A heavy burden had been lifted from my shoulders and i was secure in the knowledge that i was once again back in my true place in Her World."

"Through pampering my wife I am brought close to the center of the feminine mystery, intoxicated by it, overwhelmed by her."

"A wave of profound happiness rises in me when I worship my Goddess wife. It is heaven for me."

"I love to wash my wife's hair and scrub her in the shower, then dry her. Mostly because she loves it. If someone says it isn't important, I do not care. I know giving and loving are important to me."

"i am where i am supposed to be. i am a lucky man, and i live in the world my Mistress wants, to which She brought me. i am grateful to Her, and i tell Her so; i do my best to love, honor, and obey Her, to be as graceful as i am able in Her world."

"i prefer being immersed in my Wife's life and serving Her more than outside work and long to be the barefoot house-hubby."

And I'll end with this loving tribute posted by a most worshipful husband:

"Last night my wife fell asleep on the couch. We'd had a busy Mother's Day, which included going to a baseball game and having Chinese for dinner. I was still up... and I went over to wake her up for bed. She was asleep in a sitting position, and I knelt before her (which I often do), and wrapped my arms around her. And before I tried to wake her up, I just looked at her.

"I looked at this wonderful woman—and I thought about just how lucky I am. And I could feel the love I have for her welling up inside me as I gazed at her face. And the longer I was like this, the more entranced I felt. She was so beautiful... and I was so fortunate."

Caught in Her Perfumed Web (1.27.09)

In Chapter 5 ("Pampering and Pitching In") of my book, I describe husbands relishing giving their wives nightly footrubs and weekly (or biweekly) pedicures, then quote one such doting hubby: "My wife accused me of having a foot fetish, but I told her no, I have a wife fetish."

That certainly applies to me. My point here is that I don't think it's weird, or kinky, or even odd. I think it's actually...

Natural! We are, after all, animals (at least partly). This husband obviously agrees: "The more I served my wife orally, the more I grew to crave her scent and taste. I think now that this is natural and inevitable."

Doting husbands not only love to ogle their wives and touch them (when given the green light), and listen to them (and, yes, pay close attention), they also crave their wives' heavenly scent.

Like this devoted guy, picking up his wife's nightgown as she drops it before stepping into the adjoining bathroom: "I buried my face in her nightgown, mesmerized and intoxicated by her powerful, feminine scent. After several moments, dizzied, I finally got up and went and hung up her nightgown."

Dizzied? A married man, hyperventilating into his wife's nightgown? Yes, exactly! Listen to this guy: "I felt my sense of smell invaded by her musky aroma. I was so light headed with desire that I was prepared to do anything for her."

Or this guy, doing his wife's laundry while she's out of town on business: "I came across the outfit she wore at the office picnic, and held it to my nose and gingerly sniffed the underarms. Her fragrance and body aroma filled me and I soon had a very strong erection. Next I picked up her panties and held them to my nose and inhaled her scent from every inch of her underwear. Oh, how I missed her!"

This practice seems to be quite common among red-blooded husbands, worshipful and otherwise. Not secretly dressing up in female undergarments, but applying them as a "breathing" mask:

"For me, one of the paybacks of doing the laundry is that I get to smell her panties."

Another confession: "I find myself thinking of [my wife's] scent and taste whenever I become aroused."

A Marseillais couple I met many years ago while backpacking around Europe once told me that smell had always had been a major part of their mutual erotic attraction. They went into more detail on this than I was prepared for. (They were, after all, French.)

My wife, I have to confess, looks askance at this particular urge on the part of her loving husband. And I respect that. Other wives learn to be more laissez-faire: "Early on I admitted to my wife I sniffed Her panties on occasion. She was surprised, but pleasantly so. Which made me very happy."

And some wives can get very playful, indeed, as this husband confided to female supremacist psychologist Elise Sutton:

"After [my wife's] orgasms she removes her panties and places them inside-out on my head with the crotch right over my nose and mouth. Then I am commanded to crawl to the corner of the room for 'corner time' for 30 minutes. The whole time I am enveloped in her intoxicating scent as I have no choice but to inhale nothing but her [moist and redolent] panties plastered to my face. Her scent is so powerful and fragrant. During this time she usually watches TV or talks on the phone to girlfriends or her mother. I am in plain view of her the whole time. This whole procedure happens night after night."

Not an image of stalwart manhood, I grant you, a grown man standing in a corner, adorned in flimsy headgear. At least his penance is fragrant. There are many variations on this theme:

"Sometimes my wife rubs her panties over my face. Once she threatened that from then on I would wear her used undies the second day."

"Threatened"? How about "promised"? Many women consider the proffering of their scented panties a very special and intimate favor: "As a reward for his dutiful lovemaking, I took off my panties and gave them to him and told him to place them over his head so that the crotch was on his nose and he was looking out through the leg holes. As he followed my instructions, I explained that in time he would learn to crave my scent and taste."

Another guy, signing himself "william the submissive poet" on an female-led bulletin board, waxed lyrical on the topic:

She is wise in the ways of entrancement.
She knows the value of the gift you offer.
She has trained you to recognize Her scent
and to submit to Her spells and laughter.

One online enchantress, by-lining herself Becky, actively tutors her husband in this erotic susceptibility:

"Nose training is the process of adapting a man's nose to all [a woman's] scents and smells ... everything about a woman, including her scents, should be appealing to him. This does not come naturally to most men and therefore training is necessary. It can start with something simple, like sniffing your armpits after you finish your exercise... Once this becomes a second nature to your man, you can proceed to the next step, which could be your feet, stockings and shoes... Next will be your..."

I'll fade out there, leaving Becky's further prescriptions to the imagination, and fade in on another lady also busily enmeshing her man in her erotic web: "It amused my wife to lock me in her wardrobe among all her gorgeous clothes, leaving me surrounded in the darkness by her scented dresses."

Finally, rounding out this survey, we come to the use of milady's unmentionables as a husbandly security blanket: "My worshipful husband loves to lower himself beneath the covers to take in and savor my scent. He says it helps him to quiet his thoughts."

"On several occasions I have summoned up the courage to ask my wife if I may bring her panties to bed with me," a slightly embarrassed husband testifies. "She has, somewhat surprisingly to me, said yes. I have on those nights fallen asleep with the crotch of her panties to my nose. She knows this, and I think feels empowered by it."

It's time for final fade-out, with hubby curled up with his nightly wifely pacifier as his enchantress looks on, amused, tolerant and all-powerful:

"For some time now, I have been giving my sweet husband

the panties I wore each day, and letting him sleep with them on his pillow. He seems to really love that, and it turns me on knowing that he adores me so much. Once [when he broke one of my rules] I told him he would not be allowed to sleep with my panties. But he had made me feel so wonderful that I just couldn't bring myself to deny him for the night. I am really trying to develop a cruel streak."

Comments:
Anonymous: The more I orally serve my wife, the more I miss her taste and scent! I often fall asleep hugging her thigh... There is no better place! I feel at home and ready to obey always.

Boudoir Boys (11.14.08)

A poster on Fumika Misato's original husbands' forum playfully referred to fellow wife-worshippers who were trading tips on giving pedicures and such as "boudoir boys." In that eccentric all-male aggregation, the apparent insult was intended, and taken, as high compliment.

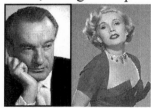

I am reminded of the late George Sanders,* an English actor (actually of Russian birth) known for his "his suave, snobbish, and somewhat menacing air" (*e.g.,* Addison DeWitt in *All About Eve*) and his celebrity marriage, back in the '50s, to Hungarian glamour queen Zsa Zsa Gabor (great aunt and prototype of Paris Hilton, another blonde famous mostly for being famous).

(* For younger readers, it was Sanders who supplied the languidly menacing voice of Kaa in Disney's *Jungle Book*, performed at a single cold reading, as I was once informed.)

No boudoir boy, Sanders is said to have been terminally annoyed when he learned, after marrying the drop-dead gorgeous actress, just how many intensive hours she required at her vanity table prior to going out.

A wife-worshipping husband, I assure you, would yield such a magnificent creature as much time as she required. Indeed, he would request a ringside seat to observe the goddess at work. He might even seek to be a "part of the process," as you will read.

As I wrote in Chapter 5 ("Pampering and Pitching In") of my book, "There are manly guys who draw their wife's bath. Who shampoo her hair. Who loofah her skin and even shave her legs. Who give facials while she luxuriates in the suds. And who are ready with a warmed, fluffed towel to enfold her as she emerges, a dripping Venus, from the bath. Who are rewarded with the further privilege of drying and powder-puffing her skin, or massaging it with moisturizing creams. And who, later, lovingly brush her hair, the traditional hundred strokes."

As one husband succinctly put it: "Through pampering my wife I am brought close to the center of the feminine mystery, intoxicated by it, overwhelmed by her."

That's about as far as you can get from the '50s-era stereotypical husband afraid of venturing into the estrogen-filled zone of milady's boudoir. But a husband can turn, or be turned, rather quickly from one type husband into the other, according to a woman signing herself "Cindy B." (in a letter to Elise Sutton's "Female Superiority" website):

"A common male complaint is how long it takes their wives to get ready and how frustrated they become having to wait. Never mind the fact that we are making ourselves beautiful for them. The male nature is an impatient nature. What men need to realize is that most of us women don't know for sure how long it's going to take, so when we say it will be five minutes, a man should not take us so literally.

"What right does a man have to bitch about how long his goddess takes to make herself beautiful? My husband would develop an attitude when my five minutes at the makeup table turned into a half-hour and I had to rush. I always felt rushed.

Now, thanks to female domination, I have rectified the situation...

"I will shower and dress in only bra and panties and call my husband into the bedroom. I put him across my lap and give him a sound spanking with my hairbrush. As I do this, I remind him that I am his goddess and that he is blessed to live with a goddess. I make him reaffirm his devotion to me and I ask me if he is going to wait patiently for me while I finish getting ready...

"By doing this I am teaching him patience. He is not permitted to watch television or get on the computer or talk on the phone. He has to sit in the chair and watch his goddess finish her hair, put on her makeup, get dressed, select her jewelry and try on different shoes. My husband is now part of the process, and I will ask him which shoes he likes the best...

"This routine has caused a real renewal in passion and romance."

Another wife accomplished almost the same result, without recourse to her hairbrush, as this ardent husband testifies: "Saturday morning after she showered, she called me in and said, 'You may watch me put on makeup and blow dry my hair if you wish.' I do love that, I have always stolen glances just to watch her do that! To me, a woman doing that is so feminine, erotic and powerful."

Both these guys are mainly there as idolators and voyeurs, though Cindy B does consult her husband's opinion on various apparel items. But some husbands are privileged to take a much more active part in "the process":

"My wife came into the bedroom and sat at her dressing table to apply her makeup. She was wearing a silk robe that I had hung in the bathroom that morning. As she applied her makeup, she noticed that there was a chip in the polish on one of her toes. 'I don't have time for a pedicure now, but fix that chip for me while I finished my makeup.' I found the polish and first cleaned the old polish from that one toe and then applied a new color and topcoat. And then I remained at her feet..."

"Do you have your husband give you a manicure and pedicure?" one matriarchal wife advises another, new to the lifestyle. "Does he blow dry your nails with his breath? Have you sent him to beauty school so he is as good as the local beautician? Do you have him run your bath, bathe you, and shave your legs? Does he warm your towels for your exit from your bath? Do you have him clean your makeup brushes and jewelry? Hand-launder your hosiery, panties and lingerie? Keep your clothes closet in order?"

Sending hubby to beauty school may seem, at first blush, far-fetched, but from the message board and newsgroup postings I've collected over the years, it seems a not uncommon occurrence.

The cosmetic arts, in fact, constitute only part of the domestic curriculum in which men are being enrolled by enterprising wives. "I have had my husband take classes in skin care, beauty and make-up, and cooking," a wife confides to Elise Sutton, "all to make his personal services better and more to my liking. He now does my nails, takes care of my hair, and does my make-up each morning."

Katherine West, a female supremacist who blogs intermittently at "Loving Female Authority," took charge of her hubby's boudoir training herself: "First he learned to bathe me, shave my legs, and paint my toe- and fingernails. Next I started teaching him how to apply my makeup and brush my hair. I allowed him to trim and shape my pubic nest. He took to his new submissive role like a duck to water."

Other anxious-to-please husbands use magazines to acquire their skill set in the feminine arts, like this enterprising individual:

"I canceled my subscriptions to *Field and Stream* and *Sports Illustrated* and replaced them with *Cosmo* and *Glamour*. I've learned about makeup, fashion, and hairstyles and patiently accompany my wife as she shops for pretty clothes, helping her pick out sexy lingerie, dresses, and heels."

Within the pseudonymous sanctuary of online FLR sites, these guys like to vie for bragging rites about which one performs the most intimate services for his queen. Some provocative examples:

"Beauty care for my wife includes bathing her, brushing hair, doing makeup and nails, laying out and assisting in dressing her."

"My Mistress requires me to massage her feet, paint her toenails and shave her legs. Occasionally she has me bathe her."

"As she sits at her dressing table blow-drying her hair, I start to massage body cream into her shoulders and back, then drop to my knees and massage her legs and feet, while she's still doing her hair. When she gets up she usually allows me a brief kiss of her pubic area followed by a quick lick of her rear. I then thank her. Oh, how I love it!"

Sounds like they get pretty carried away, doesn't it? Listen to this husband: "I'm going crazy, giving her footrubs, watching her try on new dresses, watching her put on her make-up in the morning, watching her do her fabulously thick and rich hair...."

Or this one: "I kneel next to the tub and begin to bathe my wife as I have done so many times before. I try to remain calm as I run the sponge and soap over her back, breasts and legs as she relaxes."

Well, this guy may try to remain calm, but there may be not-so-subtle visual clues to what's going on inside the kneeling bathboy, as this wife observes: "My husband gets rock hard as he bathes me."

Fdhousehusband, who used to blog at "Her Househusband's Life" and has been one of my online mentors, offers this advice to husbands embarking on wife-led marriages: "Help Her dress and undress each day."

For those Neanderthal types who presume to scold their mates for logging too much time at the dressing table, "Fd" is torn between pity and scorn:

"i always laugh when i see TV shows, films and even my male friends impatiently waiting at the door for their Wives to finish dressing and yelling out something about 'being late.' i think to myself, 'Why isn't he helping Her?' One of my important jobs is to help Her get dressed each time She heads out the door and to reverse the process when She comes home. my assistance saves Her precious minutes from Her busy day and makes myself useful. And besides, i get to enjoy this very special and intimate contact with Her!"

Another of my wife-worship mentors, Au876, obviously concurs, offering this encouragement to would-be "boudoir boys": "Fold her nightgown every morning. Make sure you clean her vanity area, her hairbrush, her hair rollers and do this every day, not just once a week. Rub her feet every night, check her toenails for rough spots and repair as necessary. A pedicure every ten days or so is not enough. Wash her stockings and hang them to dry where they are not in her way."

But I yield the last word to a woman, posting under the cyber-title of Goddess Christine: "Treat your partner like the Queen that she is. Honor her and worship her. You don't know just how lucky you are."

Comments:
Whipped One: My wife loves for me to wash her hair while she takes a bath. It is a bonding experience and a highly sensual one at that. And painting my wife's toenails is a minuscule price to pay for the wonderful gifts my wife bestows on me.

You Rang? (7.29.08)

In the posting on "Boys Night Out, Part 1" (see Chapter 12, "Degrees (and Decrees) of Domesticity"), I mention a husband whose demanding wife gave him a pager for inside the house, so she could call him on a moment's notice.

While a pager obviously does the trick, the more traditional domestic summoning device is the bell—or bells, according to one husband: "My wife placed small bells throughout the house to summon me. She didn't think this was even an unusual arrangement."

One devoted husband took the initiative and gifted his wife with a bell for a Valentine's present. "She has used and enjoyed it very much. Her eyes still twinkle each time she has a guest and picks up the bell and shakes it to summon me for some service… and it still makes me melt each time I hear it, reinforcing her superiority in an admirable way."

The bell makes an excellent gift, this husband advises, for the wife who is not yet into ruling her house and husband, giving her innocent power that she will learn to love quickly.

"Tell her that she rings the bell in your heart and that you are giving her the bell so she can signal you to come without straining her voice. Be respectful and serious and don't make a joke of it. Hopefully she will soon learn the powers she has and how they can improve her life as well as yours."

Regular use of the household handbell, according to this man's wife, demonstrates that women can and do run households and that males can be and are trained to serve their wives.

Comments:
Enoch: A bell—that's an idea. I've given my wife a very nice rolling pin as a gift (she likes to bop me on the head with it), but a bell is pretty neat. I already drop whatever I'm doing and come running whenever she calls me, but we've got three floors… Of course, my daughter has realized that I come running when my wife calls me, so she tries to imitate her voice. I can just imagine what that little stinker would do if my wife left a bell lying around.
Mark: Let me know how it works if you try it. Like the rolling pin, it can masquerade as a lighthearted, playful gift, though your wife would certainly divine the serious intent behind it, and might take to it just as she has the rolling pin. I'm filing the idea away for possible future use…
Anonymous: We have small children, so the bell doesn't work well for us. Instead I have a very small shock collar that is made for toy-size dogs. The collar and shock device is small enough to comfortably go around my balls. When my wife awakes in the morning and is ready for her breakfast, she summons me with a quick jolt.
Mark: I almost included a line or two about that method of summoning the husband—on the double!

Pecked & Whipped (4.26.08)

My father would have loved my wonderful wife, whom he never lived to see (along with his grandchildren, alas). And he would have been greatly relieved to see his younger son so well married and happy. Relieved and perhaps envious, for his troubled marriage to my mother ended in separation and bitter recrimination.

But I can't help thinking, also, at how dismayed he would be, were he still around, if he could somehow witness the secret dynamics of my marriage. The idea of a Wife-Led Marriage would have been inconceivable to a man of his generation, which accepted all the assumptions of male chauvinism as divinely ordained. That a man would have not only accepted secondary status in a marriage, but actually fostered and campaigned for that status, would be beyond his imagining.

"Henpecked and pussywhipped" might be two of the more acceptable labels he could apply to my conjugal status. Imagine a husband turning over complete financial control to his wife, indeed, abdicating the entire decision-making process in her favor! And surrendering control in the bedroom, as well. So that she decides all, and her voice is final in all matters. How could a self-respecting man let himself be reduced to such a wimpish, childlike state?

If he could see me, kneeling each night at the foot of our bed, blissfully rubbing lotion into her feet as she reads or watches TV, then kissing her feet as a concluding gesture of devotion, he would be appalled. Or what if he saw me giving her a pedicure, the painstaking care with which it is necessary to apply especially that first coat of color! What a lackey his son had been reduced to!

But then, again, might he not experience a pang of jealousy?

For he might also see the complete absence of dispute between his son and his beautiful daughter-in-law, as I acquiesce to her wishes, and even hints, in all matters. Would he not see that ours is a blissful union compared to his own?

Had he yielded to my mother, or even been susceptible to her advice, we would have held onto a particular house that went on to appreciate by many hundreds of thousands of dollars over the years that it no longer belonged to us. We would not have dissipated our family savings. My mother was frugal, my father improvident. Would we not have prospered vastly with her in control of finances? Of course we would.

And had he deferred to her, been ruled by her in all matters of disputes, our family would have stayed together.

But there are consolations, as I think back on these matters. Both my brother and I have had long and happy marriages. I don't know all the dynamics of his, so I wouldn't venture to say that his is wife-led, but I suspect that, in many areas, his wife has the deciding vote.

As well she should. Evidently my brother and I both learned a great lesson from our parents' unhappy marriage. In my case, I will say without reservation that being henpecked and pussy-whipped is a good thing for a husband to be.

Make Your Own Honey-Do List (6.4.08)

Eager to show your wife that her word is your command? Well, in all likelihood, she has issued many commands in the past that you have let slide. Perhaps because they were disguised as polite requests or even vague wishes.

Fdhousehusband, who authored the highly trafficked, but no longer extant blog, "Her Househusband's Life," describes how he finally realized this in his own marriage, and what a dramatic impact it had on him:

"i found that i was actually hindering the growth of [my Wife's] dominant side. When She would say that a light bulb was out or that there was laundry in the washer that needed to be hung up, i sometimes was too lazy to comply right away. i found that each of these actions undermined Her dominance and She would revert back to O/our old relationship. i also learned that Females speak in a diferent language. When They want something done, They don't come out and say it. In the early days, my Wife would say something like, 'My carpooler went home early so I'll be taking the bus home today.' i just accepted that like She was giving me a bit of information. What She really was saying was 'I need you to pick me up from work.' Once i understood the Female language, i learned to respond by saying things like 'May i pick You up from work today?' i found that She really responded to these 'offers' to do things for Her which She in fact had prompted with subtle 'requests.' i also think that it showed Her that i was really listening to everything She was saying."

Let's apply this seasoned advice from fd. Why not take a few moments, or as long as you need, to draw up a list of tasks that your wife has expressed even a casual interest in getting taken care of... or items she would like to have (not big-ticket items, I'm not suggesting you spend big bucks without her authorization). Not directives, but things that were perhaps dropped into the conversation in your hearing that you let slide.

Then start to work on the list, doing or buying or taking care of as many items as you can. If you do this, maybe you could let me know here, in Comment form, if your wife notices, and what the upshot is, in terms of your FLR. Positive, I hope.

By the way, I'm going to take my own—and fdhousehuband's—advice as soon as I post this and start drafting my own list, going room by room, for starters. Next time I hear her express some vague desire, I'm going to add it to my list—as a command!

Comments:
Hersforever: While I haven't done the room-by-room honey-do list, I

have started to listen for those subtle "requests" and treating them as commands—even if it's requests for me to take care of myself... and it's been very positive for her dominance.

Enoch: Early on I started carrying a little notebook and jotting down things my wife mentioned. When asked, I told her it was my "honey-do notebook." She loved it, and later replaced my little notebook with a bigger one. And then, last year, for our anniversary, she gave me a hard-backed Honey-Do Notebook.

Hersforever: Enoch - I love your idea! I think I may start doing that too, I think it would help a lot (my honey-do list tends to stay in my head, unless she writes it down for me, but I know my memory isn't perfect).

Mark: hersforever & enoch, I, too, like the notebook idea, because my short-term memory is very selective. I can remember a few things I'm interested in, like my son's baseball game times and venues, ditto for his practices. I think I'd better start cleaning up the residue of undone jobs, all those hints and mild directives she's give me in the past before I make a show of writing new ones down. Then I can produce the notebook. Except for today, which is a dedicated honey-do day, getting ready for a party for my daughter, who is graduating from 8th grade. Today I definitely need for her to write down my assignments, so I can check them off.

Enoch: I usually write down her comments into my notebook, but occasionally she will take the notebook from me and add stuff directly to it!

This topic reminds me of a tradition in the Marine Corps called "the CO's wishes." Commanding Officers learn to be careful what they say. If a battalion commander casually mentions to his Sergeant-Major that the hedges outside the battalion office needs sprucing up, you can bet that within 10 minutes there will be a working party of Marines pulled from their regular duties to do some gardening.

Mark: Enoch, the trick for me is not to spring into galvanic action, but just to get the job done, maybe when she's not looking. That way she gets accustomed to having her whims and wishes carried out like imperial edicts, but without having me making a show of instant obedience. There'll be times for that, too, but I have to pick and choose.

Anonymous: After what seemed to me like a long time of taking on every chore I could and trying to anticipate, sometimes with great success, my wife's needs, wants and whims, I found myself frustrated whenever my priorities turned out not to be my wife's priorities. And so I asked her to detail for me what my chores should be and exactly how she wanted them done. I also asked her to help me understand her personal needs better, her desires for any service that would make her life easier. To my surprise she was delighted to hear this and soon gave me a long list of chores that from then on would be my responsibility, as well as a talk about how best to serve her personal needs. Now she does only what she wants to do, while I'm doing the housework and waiting on her. Our FLR has finally come out of the closet and we are both extremely happy living out our proper gender roles.

Burnsie: I purchased a small notebook last night while running other errands for my wife. When I got home, I laid the notebook on the coffee table and she asked what the notebook was for. I said it's the honey-do notebook and explained it. You should have seen the smile on her face.

Mark: Burnsie, Anonymous, Enoch, et al., Okay, I'm convinced. I'm buying that notebook and presenting it to her, exactly as you have done. I want to see that smile.

Harnessing the Stallion (2.16.09)

Top priority for today is housework. My wife will be directing me—and helping me, since there's more to do than I could possibly get done on my own, and tomorrow we both go back to work.

I was a typical bachelor slob. Super-typical. I don't remember cleaning or dusting any of my apartments, ever. I guess I always figured if things got too bad, I'd just move.

Now, as a married man, I'm in charge of housework, in the sense of I get to do it. Just about all of it. A couple of days ago, my wife came back from Costco with a supersize bottle of Pinesol and a 2-pack of O-Cedar indoor brooms. "For you," she said.

And I love it. Well, not all the time. And not quite enough to stop writing this blogpost to get started. But I love doing the housework for her. So she doesn't have to do it.

How did this radical (and odd-seeming) conversion ever come about?

I think it must be a happy accident of evolution or creation (take your pick). Like that pronounced gap horses have between the canine teeth and the premolars; which allows for insertion of the metal bit used for controlling said horse when the animal is ridden or driven.

What is the equivalent in males of that convenient little dental slot? In a Wife-Led Marriage, it is I doubt not the established covenant giving the wife total control of when the husband will be allowed to orgasm. Though there is typically no exact correlation between how much housework is done and how often the husband is permitted climax, there is certainly a perception that the more she is pleased and pampered in every way, the more likely she will be to dispense intimate favors.

Something like that. I'll try to be more objectively precise someday, but subjectively it does feel like being in harness, with a bit in one's teeth and the reins in her hand.* That I do know and can attest to.

(*There are, of course, wife-led marriages in which the wife exercises control of her husband's sexual release by means of a male chastity device, to which she alone holds (and may even wear, locket-fashion) the only key. It is not much of a stretch to view this device, and its use by the controlling female, as akin to the equine harness-and-bit.)

And I'm sure not alone. "Husbands Who Love Housework," it sounds almost Ripleyesque, as in "Believe It or Not." Like the Portrait of Winston Churchill in a Potato Chip or a Two-Headed Llama (the pushme-pullyou of Dolittle fame).

But there are lots and lots of us who do it and love it, and love it especially when our wives don't lift a finger, except to point, or perhaps run a white-gloved digit along a shelf of knickknacks to check for dust.

Think I'm kidding? I offer in evidence a sprinkling of testimonials, culled from hundreds of the kind you can find online posted every day on Female-Led Relationship (FLR) or Wife-Led Marriage (WLM) message boards and forums.

I'll start with my old online friend, Au876, who gives proper credit to Fumika Misato for the domestication of contemporary husbands by creating her pioneering website, "Real Women Don't Do Housework":

"I am proud to be married to a Real Woman and, frankly, I don't care who knows it. I think men are much better-suited to doing the housework than women anyway.

I never felt unmanly because I worship and obey my wife...

To me there is nothing more pleasurable than serving my wife. I often find I have become sexually excited at the darnedest times. I may be ironing her clothes, cleaning the bathrooms, preparing dinner, washing dishes–you name it. And I realize I have an erection. She may not even be at home and yet I have become excited just knowing I am serving her in some fashion."

This confession, of becoming erotically aroused by repetitive domestic drudgery, is quite common, as we'll see a little farther on.

"Far from being ashamed of all the things I do for her around the house, and in the bedroom and boudoir, my greatest joy and fulfillment are to serve her with all the adoration and respect that she deserves."

"I enjoy waiting on her hand and foot."

"I am most comfortable when my fiancee chooses to relax. In our relationship, I am doing the man's work. She is not expected to lift a finger. I bring in a plate of cookies, some coffee, tea, or Perrier and we spend some time in conversation. Sometimes she is busy and I find something else to do. However, I am always on call... She goes to bed first, and I straighten up the living area. I go up to the bedroom... While the house is always neat, I only take one or two days a week to do a complete cleaning."

"I would rather she never lift a finger for domestic chores, but I have to accept her choice to pitch in. In a few years, i will retire, and i am hoping she will no longer feel the desire to pitch in and help."

"It really makes me feel good to be like say fixing her dinner while she is watching TV or napping or reading the paper. The doing of it makes me feel good and the fact that I am doing it for her makes me feel good."

As promised, here are some husbands who not only "enjoy" or "feel good" about doing housework for their wives, but get a wee bit graphic about those feelings:

"The more chores I can do for her, the more she allows me to serve her, and the hornier it makes me."

"To me, erections are a sign that our wife-led marriage is

working. I can get excited on my hands and knees, scrubbing a toilet when I think of why I'm doing it."

"The fact that I, too, may have an erection simply adds to the pleasure of washing that dish. In this way, housework can be a celebration of caring for the fine things in our home, not as a bargaining chip."

"I do get turned on sometimes doing housework but I think it is because I know I am in service to her."

"Does anybody else become aroused by doing housework? I now think about her constantly and all my housework and other chores keep me aroused as i know that i am doing them to please her. The chore has become its own reward!" (From "fdhouse-husband's" discontinued blog.)

The husbands have had their say. Now, as is only fitting, I'll cede the final word on the subject to a well-worshipped and satisfied wife:

"My husband does a lot of things for me that formerly were my chores. It was his choice to take on these responsibilities, and who am I to argue? His choice relieves me of the repetitive and tedious chores, and gives him an opportunity to demonstrate his devotion to me."

Comments:

Iowabev: I feel as comfortable with a broom or dust cloth in my hands as I do sitting at the computer writing a proposal. And when I am done cleaning the house my efforts speak for themselves.

Mark: I too enjoy the satisfaction of looking around, room by room, and seeing the floors clean, vacuumed, bathrooms shiny, clothes put away, etc. Some of this, of course, comes from the novelty of a guy doing housework. Women in WLMs must be amused by this. They've been doing this drudgery for years, with little thanks or acknowledgment. And when I'm vacuuming, I'm figuratively patting myself on the back, like "Hey, look what I'm doing, I'm vacuuming, isn't that incredible?" Kind of childish, I guess. I want to get credit for just doing it, not necessarily doing it well.

Anonymous: I love to do housework for my wife. When she is happy, I am the happiest. I think domestic servitude should be a way of life for men.

Just Do It! (6.20.08)

Another survey is out validating the findings of many previous surveys,* to the effect that husbands who apply themselves in the kitchen, laundry room and other precincts of milady's house may be rewarded by her in the bedroom.

(*According to one previous survey cited in my book, "Men who do more housework and child care have better sex lives and happier marriages than do unhelpful husbands." (Research findings published by marital researcher John Gottman, Ph.D. in the May/June 1994 issue of the *Family Therapy Networker*.))

In "Housework and Sex: What's the Connection?" released last April, University of Michigan's Institute for Social Research discovered that many housewives get turned on watching their husbands do housework.

"Sounds good," a macho husband might respond. "But is it manly? Because I wouldn't want to do anything that wasn't manly, just so I could get... well, you know."

Don't worry. You can look on housework as "Domestic Dragon-Slaying"—at least that's what I called it in my book. As I wrote in Chapter 5 ("Pampering and Pitching In"):

"A husband can step up to the plate (as it were) and be that helpmeet without endangering his masculinity (even if he dons an occasional apron). By doing so, in fact, he will be more a man in her eyes. He may even assume the radiant and transfigured status of champion—her champion. And, yes, it may pay erotic dividends down the road."

What these researchers have not yet discovered, or have not deigned to publish, however, is that it's not just wives who get turned on when husbands do housework. Husbands get turned on by themselves doing it.

Yeah, verily.

As Au876 (among many other wife-worshippers) has confessed:

"I often find I have become sexually excited at the darnedest times. I may be ironing her clothes, cleaning the bathrooms, preparing dinner, washing dishes—you name it. And I realize I have an erection. She may not even be at home and yet I have become excited just knowing I am serving her in some fashion."

I leave the "why" of this to the psychologists, normal or abnormal, to decipher. I would only point out that a male working himself up into a sexual dither in order to impress a female is not uncommon in courtship.

But for the wives, it seems, the turn-on has less to do with erotic fantasy than pragmatic reality: She's relieved and grateful to have her usually couch-bound mate up on his feet and doing some of the heavy domestic lifting, thereby lightening her burden.

"Ask any man, goes a joke I heard somewhere, and he'll tell you a woman's ultimate fantasy is to have two men at once. While this has been verified by a recent sociological study, it appears that most men do not realize that, in this fantasy, one man is cooking and the other is cleaning."

Another old joke to the same purpose: "What's the sexiest thing a young dad can do for his wife?" Answer: "The dishes."

That's not to say that women can't indulge some wild fantasies in regard to domestic arrangements. Take this sampling of responses by young women to an Internet survey question, "What would your dream househusband do for you?"

"Keep my house spotlessly clean and have delicious meals prepared for me every night—and dress up when I want to go out!"

"Do laundry, pay bills, walk the dog, run errands, and have dinner waiting on the table for me at night naked!"

"Keep the refrigerator full ...cook, clean & kiss me as I walk in the door."

"Fetch my book, hold my bookmark, and rub my feet whilst I read."

"Pick up our kids, help them with homework, and be happy to see me!"

And this final fantasy: *"He'd have my period for me."*

The female-led nature of this domestic setup was also made explicit by several women who responded to the "dream house-husband" survey, to wit: *"I want a man who truly understands the business of maintaining home & family and who understands in no uncertain terms I am the CEO."*

The message to married males I can sum up by adding three words to the tagline of this blog, i.e.: "If you want your wife to be a goddess, worship her… and serve her!"

What Have You Done for Her Lately? (4.29.08)

My bachelor pad was a pigsty. Do people still use that word? It's more descriptive, I think, than pigpen. No, I didn't use empty pizza boxes as room dividers, but there were archaeological layers of clutter, and the kitchen floor and ceiling and walls and appliances were all coated with fried hamburger grease.

Flash forward a couple decades, and you'll find me sweeping floors, vacuuming, spraying 409 on every visible surface, making beds, ironing, picking up junk, folding my wife's nightgown and lovely unmentionables, cleaning up after the kids, endlessly, scraping sugary goo off the coffee table. I don't do much dusting, but maybe I'll get there.

What worked the one-eighty change in me, from domestic slob to wannabe Mr. Clean?

Wife worship worked the miracle, of course. It didn't happen overnight, but after a few years of effort, it's pretty much crystallized from intention into daily habit, even when I'm not actively thinking about helping my wife, or making her life easier. I could do much more, and intend to, but I'll give myself an attaboy for how far I've come. And my wife "brags on me," too, as Au876 used to say.

"The more you do for your wife, the more you want to do," insists one devoted husband, "and the more you want to do, the more you discover things you can do. It just grows." (Quoted in Chapter 5, "Pampering & Pitching In," of my book.)

That's not all that grows on these domestically devoted husbands. As A876, wrote: "I may be ironing her clothes, cleaning the bathrooms, preparing dinner, washing dishes—you name it. And I realize I have an erection. She may not even be at home and yet I have become excited just knowing I am serving her in some fashion."

Is that kinky or what? And yet, this benignly delusional behavior results in a clean house and a happier wife. My advice to husbands just taking up the renewed courtship of their wives?

Go thou and do likewise.

Ask your wife for how-to hints and helps. Or check out Fly-Lady.Net or Jeff Campbell's Speed Cleaning. And start slaying her domestic dragons on a daily basis.

Men at Work (12.10.09)

Q: I get the "perpetual courtship" thing—treating the wife like a queen, flowers, chocolates, love notes, etc. And getting down on my knees to give her footrubs, even pedicures, can be a real turn-on. But I don't buy into the courtship angle of doing more and more of the housework, even including dusting and ironing. You can call it "domestic dragon-slaying" if you like, but that doesn't make it manly.

A: Well, you certainly sound more macho than I am. And in my much younger, studlier days, the only apron I wore was a leather nail apron as a rough-framing carpenter (or carpenter's helper). But these days, yes, in my daily romantic service to my wife, I make the bed, fold her nightgown, iron her blouses (along with my shirts), and, yes, even dust knickknacks. I've even surrendered the remote (though I sometimes do my domestic chores listening to baseball, football and basketball on a headset radio).

The challenge remains, can a guy follow all the steps of wife worship, including "doing more and more of the housework," without sacrificing his masculinity and self-respect?

My answer is yes, unless he *wants* to be emasculated, or his wife wants him to be emasculated. Instances of this apparently abound—where men dress, or are dressed, in French maid costumes and go teetering about in high heels and makeup, feather duster in manicured hand.

But, judging by all the FLR accounts I've seen from husbands and wives over many years, this aspect of role reversal is definitely in a marginalized minority

I suggest that most wife-trained husbands perform their domestic duties in a no-frills, masculine fashion. As one of my favorite oracles, Au876, once wrote in Lady Misato's original Wife Worship Forum:

"Over the years my wife has pointed out that men are better suited for housework in a lot of different ways. Men are stronger (generally) and thus more able to move furniture so you can vacuum or sweep. Men have more upper body strength and thus are more suited to scrubbing, mopping, etc. Men are taller and can more easily reach up to clean high places... Men don't have to worry about breaking a nail or messing up nail polish while they are cleaning and are not nearly as concerned about how their hands look. She makes good points and I totally agree with her."

Of course, Au adds that "the main reason I do all the housework is because she wants me to."

Get the image of the hunky helpmate? One of the gurus of housework online, Jeff Campbell, seems to fit the manly matrix (oops, wrong term there!). On his website, Jeff sells a very manly looking apron, even if it doesn't have belt loops for power equipment and a 20 oz. waffle-patterned framing hammer. "Professional cleaners dress for the job in comfortable, washable clothing designed for work," Campbell writes. "Check out their supportive shoes and kneepads. Goggles and gloves protect against chemicals."

And, yes, some of those henpecked, pussywhipped husbands "hoovering" the carpets and "swiffering" the linoleum are imposing dudes, well equipped for domestic dragon-slaying. Here's a trio:

"My husband is a strong-willed man who enjoys much control and leadership in his field," a wife brags on Lady Misato's website. "He is 6-3 while I am barely 5-5, yet, I even dominate him physically as he does not resist my pushing and pulling on him... He is much happier and is often humming or singing around the house now."

No. 2 sounds even more macho: "I am six feet four inches tall, I played college football, I can still bench press over 300 pounds, and I have a black belt in karate. I could kick most guys' asses, if I were not such a loving and peaceful guy. My wife is a petite woman who weighs about one third of what I do and who is eight years younger than I. Yet she rules my life to the maximum. She is the bossiest and most dominant female I have ever met and I am madly in love with her."

Here's our third tough guy: "In terms of my own manliness, I am a few months away from being a black belt in karate, I am the father of two almost grown children, own a successful business, and am in a romantic blissful relationship with a fantastic woman. I have given my Mistress Wife the reins to our relationship, not because I am a wimp, but out of a choice."

Macho or not, what about a fair division of household chores? As I wrote in Chapter 5, "Pampering and Pitching In," of my book, "In today's two-income marriages, ought the woman be expected to tie on an apron the minute she parks her briefcase at the front door?... Shouldn't the husband voluntarily turn off the Big Game du Jour and lend a hand? Of course he should. He should, in fact, let his work-weary wife log a few hours of her own in the La-Z-Boy with a magazine and a Merlot."

There is knightly satisfaction in keeping Milady's castle spotless, as this husband relates on Lady Misato's site: "I do most of the housework now. I don't consider this a chore but a pleasure. I owe her so much and love her so much that I enjoy doing everything I can. I listen, respond, obey, and love every minute of it."

He is also likely to be romantically rewarded for all his domestic drudgery, as this leading wife makes plain: "If you want to pamper a woman, do the housework for her. Do you think a woman likes to come home in the evening and do housework while her husband is watching tv and drinking beer? Having a husband who willingly does all the housework, laundry, etc., is a daily pampering. A woman loves to be pampered. Don't ever forget that."

A CNN online article last June highlighted this issue, a familiar one in Wife-Led Marriags, in an article titled "Housework and sex: What's the connection?"

It begins: "Jen Simmons loves to watch her husband Danny tend to their two little boys, mop the floor or hang a picture. She also finds it sexy. Men do more housework than they used to, a study says, although they create more of it." And goes on: "I am very turned on when he's doing housework," says the 36-year-old Camden, Delaware resident, a middle school teacher."

Here are some supporting testimonials from houseworking hubbies:

"Before our FLR, we fought about housework constantly. Now I truly have learned to enjoy it. I enjoy pleasing Her. She especially loves it when I clean the toilets. It makes Her frisky. And I like a frisky Wife!"

Cautionary Note: Husbands shouldn't expect a romantic payoff for substandard housework. As one Loving Female Authoritarian puts it, "I don't want to find panties or socks inside out or folded sloppy. Watch out if I do. I have become much more demanding as the relationship has grown."

"It is a proven fact that most men cannot or will not clean as well as a woman," another female head-of-house states, "but a little known fact is they can be taught!"

Comments:

Bob: Many of my blue collar friends are more likely to do most or all of the housework in their marriages than my friends that work in an office. If you have been swinging a 10 lb sledgehammer all day long, no one is going to think that you are a wimp for taking off your toolbelt when you get home and putting on an apron. Also a blue collar guy often judges his worth not by how much money he earns, but by how hard he works and how useful he is.

Anonymous: I'm kind of astounded that any FLR-aspiring man wouldn't understand the correlation between housework and romance. Because the wifely burden of neverending laundry, dishes, cooking, and cleaning is the exact opposite of an aphrodisiac. Truly.

But does this mean we want our men to abdicate their manliness? No way! My boyfriend is a civil engineer. Loves sports, working on cars, pumpin' iron, and grillin' on the barbie. A guy's kinda guy. And he is just as hot cleaning the toilet (which I hate doing) as he is changing a tire. His status as sole toilet cleaner has only raised his desirability in my eyes. He's happy to save me from something I detest. And I adore him for it.

Anonymous No. 2: My wife and I mutually made the decision that I would be doing all of the housework when we began out WLM 6 years ago. Now I prepare most of our dinners, do the wash and iron many of her clothes. She loves it! She makes me clean the house wearing only my shorts and she teases me by walking around or watching TV when I clean wearing only bra and panties. Every so often the bra will come off...

Proud to Serve (12.29.09)

I hope my readers have been having, and are continuing to have, restful and rewarding holiday times. Okay, I just wrote "restful" because it's alliterative, but what could I be thinking? "Hectic but happy" is more like it for most of us.

I haven't had time to post, or do much else, with all the last-minute shopping and returning and light-stringing (we go nuts) and cruising for the last *&%$#!* mall parking place. But I'd better post something before you all wander off—especially since the blog counter not long ago rolled over to 200,000 page views.

So here are a few words about what "john," a female-worshipping blog colleague, calls "submissive pride." As he succinctly puts it:

"Men who are submissive—and proud of it—should be free to identify themselves as such and not worry about what others think. I'm a strong secure submissive man who thinks bowing to the authority and command of a strong dominant woman makes sense and is the right choice for me."

The first time I encountered a husband openly boasting of his devoted and submissive service to his wife was about ten years ago, on Lady Misato's original Wife Worship husbands' forum. The mainstay of that forum, Au876, wrote often of how proud he was to cater to his wife's wishes, even in front of others, as in this example:

"We went to visit some of my wife's girlfriends at a lake cabin a couple of years ago. We had to take our own sheets and etc. One of the first things I did after getting the car unloaded was to make up our bed and put her clothes away. Later we were all sitting around talking. My wife asked me 'Have you made up my bed yet?' One of the ladies started to laugh like that was a stupid thing to expect of a man. But I quickly responded telling her yes and I had hung up all of clothes too…

"My wife was real proud of me. The lady who laughed made some sort of comment about what a good husband I was, and my wife responded saying something like, 'He knows what is expected of him.'

"I was not embarrassed. I was proud of myself. I had done what I was supposed to do. The fact my wife asked me was a sure sign she did not intend to keep my status a secret from them. The fact I had already done it was a sure sign to her I was not ashamed of my status… Even when others notice, I am proud to treat my wife as my Queen."

Has the social stigma of appearing henpecked and pussy-whipped lessened any over the past decade? Maybe not. But certainly more and more guys in the FLR lifestyle are speaking out proudly, like this:

"I used to be ashamed or would hide it. If I was ironing, I

would act like it wasn't me ironing. The same with laundry or cleaning. I've since grown up and said 'you know what, I should be proud of helping out' and I've stopped worrying about what others think. I beam with pride when someone makes a comment about how great my wife is treated."

"Some people may look at our lifestyle and say we are hen-pecked. As for myself, I'm proud to serve and please my wife. I also think it's great to have a sense of humor about these things."

"I felt really good doing the housework. I felt happy knowing how pleased my wife would be, and I felt kind of proud of my-self for being so productive."

Here, from the Spouseclub Archives, is a young guy bursting with pride over his upcoming marriage to "a very high-powered partner in a large law firm." She proposed to him, natch, and he still sounds giddy about being swept up in her orbit and at his impending role as her devoted househubby:

"I am so proud of her and her accomplishments and I would do anything to make sure that her needs are taken care of and that our lives run smoothly... I read in a post here about the hus-band taking the wife's name. I would be so proud to have her name."

A female Spousechatter strongly seconds that idea: "Today a man who takes his wife's name can do so with pride and respect for his wife's status and accomplishments."

For all these guys, accepting and openly acknowledging their innately submissive side constitutes an "out-of-closet" experi-ence, a first step toward psychological liberation that needs and deserves to be encouraged.

"You were probably born with the trait of submissiveness," writes the female webmaster at Caring Domination to a submis-sive male seeking her advice. "You want to please others. That's good. You probably submit to a higher moral code, which is very good... Be proud of your submissiveness. You are a caring person who could make a wonderful husband."

For a few men, "submissive pride" seems to come naturally. An example is this guy, who brags about being raised in a strongly matriarchal home: "I am proud to say that I have been Female Led my entire life. My Mother (a strong beautiful woman) made sure I respected women and understood a woman's powers and that I was accepting of female leadership."

But for most men to accept their own submissiveness is not an easy step, and to "out" themselves proudly before others is harder still. Often it takes the strong, helping hand of a Loving Female Authoritarian to facilitate this important psychological rite of passage. Understandably. As Kathy, who writes the "Femdom 101" blog, explains. "Many of the submissive men who blog, or email to me feel ashamed of their status. A woman needs to learn to build up her man, to praise him for things he does good, to encourage him to be a better servant."

She praises one of her female commenters for doing exactly this: "It sounds like Bella is perfect at this. Her husband still has an ego, but the source of his male pride has been changed. A quick little comment from Bella about what a good servant her husband is, and he beams with pride. It is especially pleasing since she made the remark in front of female friends. Bella's husband may be a slave, but she still managed to put him on a pedestal."

Kathy's observation about changing the source of a male's pride by praising him in front of "female friends" for being "a good servant" is the precise tactic recommended in a recent article on the "DreamLover Labs" site by Kathrin Cohen.

The article is humorously couched in psychological jargon, titled "Identity Reframing: Pride and Shame as Powerful Means of Behavior Control." But the author loses no time in getting down to brass tacks. "Make him proud to serve," Ms. Cohen tells her female readers, "make it clear to your male that his submission is bettering him and is something to be proud of":

"It goes without saying that, given the many beneficial effects, you should aim at letting everyone know about your male's obedience. Create a formidable reputation which he will be afraid of ruining by being rude or uppity. Present him as the most helpful, well mannered man you have ever met.

"As the male learns to fight to preserve his reputation as the 'most obedient,' 'most attentive' husband, or the 'boyfriend who never ever talks back to you,' something important will happen. The male will begin to associate his sense of pride to the quality of his service, which is key to long-lasting obedience."

Ms. Cohen concludes her article: "You are sending a clear message to your male's subconscious that: serving females is good; everyone thinks so; you love him for it; people expect it of him; he's good at it; so he should be very proud of it."

Think no guy would allow himself to be so nakedly manipulated by women for their own ends? You'd be wrong. Here's one guy, for instance, who takes the manipulative bait, hook, line and sinker: "My willingness to obey and do any chore [for my girlfriend, her sister and daughter] to increase their time together relaxing, has earned me the title of being well trained, which I love to hear. Just a few words of encouragement from these superior females and I feel rewarded and refreshed."

"Ms. Barbara," who moderates a provocative FLR group on Yahoo!, is another enthusiastic proponent of Identity Reframing—transforming male submissive shame into male submissive pride. As she writes:

"I want [my husband] to be proud to be a trained pussy eater and worshipper. Pride and submissiveness are no contradiction. He manages to make me happy and I think that he's got a right to be proud of that. That is the kind of pride every man should strive for, i.e., making a woman happy, first and foremost, before his own satisfaction and pleasure."

A wife wishing to show off her man's dutiful status, as Ms. Cohen recommends, but lacking a female confidante, may urge hubby to reveal his submissiveness online, as in this note to Elise Sutton:

"Ms Sutton, my wife is thrilled with the changes in our marriage. She is proud of what she has accomplished and she wanted me to share our story." One suspects this husband shares his wife's pride in his accomplishments and has bought into the new self-image she has helped to shape.

But is it really that simple? By acting proud of her devoted male, even bragging about him to her girlfriends, can a clever wife really transform her man's embarrassment and shame to submissive pride, and a resolve to be even more devoted to her service?

The answer seems to be yes. The oft-quoted Au876 swells with pride whenever his wife "brags on him" to her girlfriends. For him there is no greater reward. "I am proud to be known to do her bidding," he states flatly. "There is no dishonor in making the bed, cleaning the house, shopping for groceries, cooking the meals, washing the clothes. That is the way a husband should be." Likewise, on the Spouseclub Archives, Charles (aka Mr. Lisa), confides to Ms. Lynda that every day one of his main motivations is to do everything he can to "make Lisa proud of me."

"I want my wife to be proud of me in my service and devotion to her," echoes another worshipful husband.

But what of the wife? Is bragging about a submissive husband merely a clever manipulative tactic to "reframe his identity"? Can a wife truly be proud of a husband who grovels before her on a daily basis, seeking only to do her bidding?

The answer, again according to Mistress Kathy, is emphatically yes. Women often ask her how she can be proud of her husband, when his status in the marriage and the household is so drastically reduced. The answer, she asserts, "is that I am proud of him for all the sacrifices he makes for me. I am proud of him for living his life according to my rules and priorities. This is not easy for a man, but he does a wonderful job of it... He may not be a man's man in the John Wayne tradition, but he is every bit a man."

Or, as Au876 once put it, he is every bit "her man."

Seen in this light, the groveling husband becomes his wife's loyal and loving knight, bending his knee to signal his devoted service. This aspect of male submissive as romantic gallantry is also touched on by Kathrin Cohen in her semi-playful article on "Identity Reframing": "Though concepts of chivalry are by some considered obsolete, they still resonate strongly with most males."

"Men are capable of tremendous service and sacrifice when we are truly committed to a goal," wrote an anonymous and extremely articulate wife-worshipper years ago. "We are most content when we have a great adventure before us. We have that cause at the feet of our Goddesses. To lift them to their rightful roles as the divine inspiration to our otherwise sad and empty lives. To give our bodies, our minds and our lives to serve and defend these brave, beautiful, nurturing, challenging, life-giving, playful, wondrous women. With their guidance, our lives once again become real and connected to the natural world."

Amen, brother!

Comments:

Anonymous: I loved this post. It really resonates with what women want, and I'm sure that if more guys took that sort of approach, femdom would proliferate crazily. Your wife is a lucky woman.

Worship Her: My wife's friends all have seen how well she is treated and they have asked her how she does it. She has told them straight out that we have a WLM and that I am totally obedient to her and must please her any way she tells me to. Plus, she told them, I must do things to please her every day without being told. Her friends now know that I do all of the housework, laundry, most ironing and much of our cooking. I know her friends have taken her advice and 2 of them now have a WLM with their husbands. Mark, my wife and I read every one [of your posts].

Runpb: I'd like to encourage all the readers who have not read Mr. Remond's book to purchase and read it. Then you can read it to your wives! Build a date night around THAT concept!

Bob: I am always puzzeled by guys who want to lead a WLM lifestyle but are scared that people will find it strange. I am not married but when i have dinner at a woman's house i usually clean up afterwards and do the dishes. I have yet to find someone who thought that a man doing dishes is strange.

6

MAXIMUM EXPOSURE

Male Cluelessness (4.21.08)

"Women generally want men 'to just know' without having to be told." The quote is from radio talk-show host Dennis Prager, and it resonates with me as true. Prager goes on (as quoted on p. 58 of my book): "But the vast majority of men do not 'just know.' We rarely have a clue. That is why women often think of their man as 'clueless.' But cluelessness in this area is not a male fault; it is a male trait."

This works as a generalization, I think, applicable to almost every aspect of male-female relations. But, for the sake of blog-post brevity, let's narrow the focus a bit. Guys rarely detect the next emotional land mine in the terrain ahead until they step on it and are blown sky-high.

How many times, especially in the bad old days before I launched my wife-worship campaign, did I find myself blind-sided by such a domestic detonation? Here was my darling, out of the blue, angry or tearful or deeply troubled over something that completely eluded me.And I, by omission or commission, was somehow the cause.

And I was, of course, completely clueless.

It still happens, I confess. Despite my efforts at vigilance, keeping a lookout posted ahead for the slightest squall in her

116

emotional weather, I still find myself occasionally unprepared. But the frequency of serious blowups is much less, and my wife is much more apt to give me credit for daily diligent attention to her needs and moods and consistent attempts to keep the court-ship going.

That's why I prescribe perpetual courtship. A husband dare not define the status of his marriage as safely "quo" and his bride permanently wooed and won. Far better to treat marriage like one of those emergency preparedness drills, in which the husband must go through a daily checklist of essential tasks, with his wife's happiness ever before him as the objective to be secured.

What can he do today to further that objective? What ought he not to do?

Is that overdoing things? No, it isn't. Male cluelessness is endemic and insidious. And marriage is a daily crisis. Define it otherwise and a husband is asking for the next crisis to fall on his clueless head.

A final word, from the Introduction of my book: "Courtship and reconciliation are clearly defined crises in a man's life. He will do anything to win the woman of his dreams; should he lose her, he will do anything to win her back. Why, then, is he not willing to do anything, on a daily basis, to keep her contented? Because husbands don't perceive that a wife can be lost if never again wooed or won, that marriage is also a crisis, deserving of extreme efforts. This is not punishment, but reward: His wife is more than worthy of the very best he can give."

Curbing My Enthusiasm, Part 1 (12.2.08)

Pretty much I'm a quiet guy, shy in social situations. But every once in a while, who knows why, out pops Jack-the-Chatterbox, not listening to or simply talking over others, including my wife, in my eagerness to blurt out my next bon mot. Could be a quip. Could be something better left unsaid.

There's that baggy-pants guy with the squirting selzer bottle again, high-stepping across the stage through the spotlight. Get the hook.

My wife has seen this act many times before. She may boot me in the shins under the table at the time, or rebuke me later in the car. She may let it pass.

I'm not as incorrigible as I used to be, Lord knows. Over the years I've tried to keep a lid on what Alan Greenspan (in another context) termed "irrational exuberance." Way back in elementary school, I was one of those first-one-with-the-answer kids, like the "grade-grubbing," precocious girl "Summer" in the movie *School of Rock*.

But, clearly, I can still act like that attention-seeking second-grader.

Wife worship—serious wife worship, the kind that evolves into a committed wife-led marriage—offers me a chance to finally outgrow this juvenile behavior.

In fact, on the various wife-worship and female-led message boards and forums, you will find many husbands struggling with this kind of conversational boorishness, in order to show greater respect for their leading wives. Here is an example of a guy sharing some New Year's Resolves:

"I will not back talk to my wife. I will not interrupt. I will not comment on everything. I will listen carefully so she does not have to repeat things. When she says to stop something that is annoying her, I will stop immediately, no whining, no moping, no bad attitude. I will not disagree with her in public."

As I wrote in my book (Chapter 6, "Being Known by Her"): "I mean, really, how can you worship your wife if you won't even stop and listen to her? If you can't turn down the volume of your own thoughts and preoccupations long enough for her voice to get through to you?"

Another husband offers a few conversational specifics: "Yes, we need to watch what we say. In private, it is best to listen more and speak less. Consider her feelings, answer her questions directly and honestly, be open about your emotions and pay attention to her verbal and non-verbal clues. In public, show deference to her ideas and views, do not interrupt or use foul language. She will love it if you stand up for her opinions."

"I make it a practice to sit and listen with total focus to whatever my wife is saying," recommends another husband.

I came up with almost identical advice in my book: "Now when my wife speaks, even offhandedly, a little bell rings, reminding me, 'This is not background noise, this is the woman you love and adore.' Especially if she speaks in a tone that signals she really need my attention, I stop—whatever I'm doing. If I'm standing, I often sit down, to concentrate on what she's saying."

But I especially like this prescription for husbandly comportment posted on the old Spouseclub message board by a "Mr. Louise," describing his matriarchal home:

"My greatest thrill in our social life is when we have a few friends over and the wives all talk openly to each other and the men are finally lulled by Ms. Louise's dominance and their own wives into quiet, sensible submission. The sound of male quiet during female conversation is the music of a matriarchal home. If I excitedly offer my opinion Ms. Louise often returns me to my place with a loving chide: 'Honey, please, the women are speaking now.' And that is the motto of our matriarchy: the women are speaking now; men, you've had your chance, and please be silent."

Curbing one's conversational excesses is obviously more difficult lacking a no-nonsense wife like Ms. Louise, or this authoritarian wife: "In my home, my husband is forbidden to interrupt the feminine talk, nor to command any conversation, except with my explicit consent."

At our house, I have to do the self-scolding, or self-reminding: Don't give her the benefit of your opinions on everything, don't sound off or weigh in before she has a chance to speak. Find out what she thinks.

And don't, for heaven's sake, interrupt her. No matter how much you feel compelled to share some cosmic thought. Don't interrupt if she's on the phone, or chatting with someone, including our kids, or reading a book, or watching TV. Unless the sky is genuinely falling.

In other words, respect what she's doing. Let your urgency wait. And don't just stand there, silently importuning. Back out of the room, go away, try again later.

As this wife counsels, "My hubby learned that when he got 'the look' while I was working on a project that it was best for him not to interrupt but to find something else to do—fast."

So, what I do with my conversational enthusiasm these days is—blog! I've got a bit more to say on this topic, but I'll save it for Part 2.

Curbing My Enthusiasm, Part 2 (12.10.08)

Actress Marlo Thomas recalled how annoyed she would get when her husband, TV perennial Phil Donahue, would walk into their bedroom and demand in his resonant on-air voice, "Honey, where are my shoes?"

What annoyed her the most, Thomas recalled, was not her husband interrupting her with this childish demand, but that she always knew exactly where he had left his size-12 wingtips.

Apparently even celebrity wives are used to playing mommy to childish husbands, used to being interrupted with self-centered, impatient, even infantile demands—"Find my shoes," "Tie my tie," "Sew my button," "What happened to my leftover pepperoni slice?"

It's true, our wives *do* know everything, including where we left our wallet, our shoes, our car keys, our cell phone. But barging in on the wife with me-first demands, derailing her train of thought, not respecting whatever activity, or inactivity, she may be engaged in—these are emphatically not courtship behaviors.

Knocking on Heaven's Door

So knock it off, guys! But do knock—if you do need to speak to her and she has closed the bedroom door. Never barge in, Lord of the Manor-style.

In many wife-led marriages, this is pretty standard protocol, as per this message board sequence (on which I have altered names):

George: "Do other guys have to knock on the bedroom door, before they are allowed in? My wife now insists that I knock before I can enter. Recently on holiday in a villa we rented with the rest of the family I didn't knock and she wanted to know why. I said I didn't want anyone to know I had to knock first, and she replied that she didn't care and I was to knock in future. Sometimes she lets me in and other times she refuses until she finishes changing. I have to wait at the door until it's my turn to change. This makes me feel how much she is in control."

Wife No. 1: "I agree, you shouldn't automatically enter when you feel like it. I don't much like being interrupted unexpectedly either. It also places you in a 'asking' mindset before barging in. It tells you that you are NOT in control in the bedroom, SHE is! If others ask you about it, you can say, 'My wife asked me to not unexpectedly open the door with other people in the villa, and I respect her wishes.' Then you sound like the most thoughtful man around."

Wife No. 2: "You sound very thoughtful - Keep up the good service. Just knock in all situations and neither one of you will have to give it much thought."

Wife No. 3: "Of course you should knock on her bedroom door, George. When my sweet hubby brings me my morning tea, or at other times he wishes to enter, he always knocks first and does not enter until I say so."

George: "Thank you for replying, ladies. I'm glad I am not alone."

One More Step

Not interrupting one's spouse is a good first step in wife worship. But some husbands, practicing perpetual courtship, take it a step farther… letting themselves be interrupted by their wives.

As I wrote in my book (Chapter 6, "Daring to Be Known by Her"): "If this seems a bit extreme, remember, I'm trying to alter lifelong habits, and it's not easy. And, anyway, isn't this the kind of attention that a spouse deserves?... Most important, isn't this the way you listen to someone you're madly in love with?"

The answer is emphatically "Yes!"—at least according to this "Amen Chorus" of dutiful husbands:

"Allow yourself to be interrupted."

"When she speaks now, or asks for my attention for something she wants to tell me, or even off-handedly, I don't give her half an ear."

"Whenever your wife says something to you, stop what you're doing and listen up. Don't overdo, don't be servile, but pay careful attention."

"I might be reading a book or doing whatever, but when my wife speaks, I immediately attend to her."

"I really, really want to pay attention to her every word. When she does make a request of me, I treat it as a command. I have no sense of a mental debate in my mind like I have in the past."

"My wife isn't all that bossy but when she has something to say, I listen, and when she even hints at something for me to do, I do it."

In some female-led households, of course, the wife is encouraged to be more than a bit bossy. One such matriarchal wife instituted the following conversational rule for her mate: "If I speak, you must be silent, even if you are speaking first."

Comments:
Her man: This is awesome! I am a male that is trying to find ways to be more submissive and have my wife become more dominant. Knocking on the bedroom door is such a great idea. It gives her total control over the bedroom. Thank you for the tip.

Mark: Agreed. In some of those quoted instances, I omitted the not irrelevant fact that the wife had taken possession of the bedroom and the husband now slept elsewhere. But more commonly, I think it works in the normal shared bedroom, respecting the wife's privacy, and primacy, if you like. In our house, she closes it mostly because of the kids, but almost always I respect that and knock.

John: What a simple and powerful way to assert a power differential and make a relationship more mindful! And, of course, there is usually a long way to go in this regard just to get back somewhere near 50:50, much less tilt it to her favor.

Mark: True enough what you say about getting back to 50-50. My wife is extremely considerate, so I relish the times when she is... oh, shall we say, just a bit peremptory with me?

Carousel: I love the idea of letting her interrupt me—stop talking as soon as she starts talking, even if I was talking first. I notice that we've had fights where she interrupts me. Now I'll just let her interrupt me. It's a subtle thing she may not even recognize—just have a feeling that I'm generally being more cooperative.

Pillow Talk — Give it a Try, Guys (6.27.08)

Have you noticed? We seem to have come a long way from the "strong, silent type" mold of Hollywood heroe like Wayne, Coop, Clint, *et al.* Vince Vaughan, Shia LaBeouf, Adam Sandler, even Robert Downey Jr. as Iron Man—who am I forgetting?—these guys tend to talk a blue streak. In fact, you can't shut 'em up.

Yet the real macho guy, master of the one-syllable repartee (or grunt), remains the archetype. Especially in the bedroom. It's the girl who cries out, "Oh, James!" While Bond just gives a tomcat shrug and arches an eyebrow.

This silent gunfighter image has had a lasting effect on generations of guys. We strive to underplay our speaking parts before, during and after sex. Whatever you do, don't show your emotions. It's embodied in today's casual sex hookups.

But this manly protocol gets chucked right out the window in an FLR (female led relationship), or WLM (wife led marriage). And if it doesn't, it should.

The goal here, of course, is not to hide one's worshipful feelings from one's beloved, but to reveal them. Don't try to be the "strong, silent type" when it comes to your adoration and devotion.

In Chapter 6 ("Daring to Be Known by Her") of my book, I quote Fumika Misato:

"Consider a true and honest confession of your feelings to your wife. Express yourself without reservation. Don't be afraid to let your wife know how powerful she is. Her primary goal is to get your attention, and all that entails. Let her know that she has it. And she will be impressed, even touched, by your honesty."

Lady Misato goes even farther, recommending wives get their husbands to tell them everything, every night (she recommends the marriage bed as the site for these nightly confessions).

While Lady Misato instructs wives in ways to extract these nightly confessions and avowals of love from their mates, there's nothing wrong with a husband initiating them.

For instance, during lovemaking. Again, to quote my book:

"For me, the throes of conjugal sex tend to trigger impromptu, lovestricken confessions. The most impassioned avowals suddenly populate my brain—mostly unoriginal, even trite. I used to suppress these, trying to maintain at least a semblance of manly reserve, knowing my blurted words might sound embarrassing afterward.

"I no longer do that—muzzle myself... These days, during the final crescendos of passion, I am more likely to let myself go—verbally as well as seminally. My wife has heard me stutter out empurpled phrases like, 'I'm so lucky to be married to you.' Or: 'You are my queen.' Or: 'I love you, I love you, I love you.' Or: 'I want to belong to you completely.' Not a few times I have reverted to simply repeating her name over and over and over, mantra-like."

Okay, afterwards I sometimes feel a wee bit embarrassed. How must all that have sounded to her? Was I gushing like a lovesick schoolboy?

Maybe. But the point is, I'm *not* Clint Eastwood or John Wayne. I'm not *muy macho*. You won't see me leaving the gal of my dreams as I ride off alone into the sunset on my favorite horse. As I wrote:

"I *do* want to belong to her completely, etc., etc., and I want her to know it, to know me. What I have given voice to really are the innermost secrets of my heart—things I want to share with my beloved."

My wife, as it happens, is not a talker. She's the strong silent type in our marriage. She has not commented on my confessional binges during lovemaking, neither praised nor scolded me for them. They are just kind of "out there," on the record. Because I cannot help myself, I have to tell her everything.

Another instance of FLR role reversal.

Comments:
Enoch: My wife is also the one who is less likely to express her feelings. She loves to talk—conversation is important to her—but she rarely talks about her feelings. I am the one who constantly tells her how much I love her and how lucky I am. She accepts it, but doesn't elaborate on it.
Susan's Pet: You can still be a hero's hero, yet worship and serve your partner. My point is, there is no typical role for the submissive man to play. We may have some common traits, but we are all different.

Pillow Talk & Pillow Moans (6.30.08)

This is a postscript to the preceding post about another kind of role-reversal behavior observed in FLRs. Namely, that husbands are starting to gasp and moan and vent their emotions during the climactic moments of lovemaking.

Some husbands are being encouraged, or even manipulated by their leading wives into opening up in this way. Other husbands simply find themselves unable to suppress this unmacho behavior—or feel that they no longer have to suppress it, after years of doing so.

An interesting discussion of this behavior, from both sides of the bed. appeared on the well populated FLR message board, SheMakesTheRules.Com (an outgrowth of Barbara Abernathy's Venus on Top Society). Perhaps the board ops won't mind if I pass on a few snippets from the several provocative responses:

A woman posts: "And just as men love to hear a woman moan and make noise, we love hearing that kind of feedback from men. At least I do! I L-O-V-E to hear a man moan, groan, and cry out when making love... It comes across as positive feedback. and lets me know that my partner is most definitely into the moment!"

Two women echo this sentiment:

"I completely agree a 100%. And the thing is, if we are in a situation where I just want silence and he's talking, or I want him to tell me exactly what he's feeling and all I'm getting are moans, I tell him what to do!"

"I love it when my lover moans, talks, shakes and loses control! I like to know that I am in total control of his pleasure and climax, after I have been satisfied of course. I also love to hear that he is mine... all mine to do with what I wish."

A husband confesses: "My wife loves for me to make sounds in bed—she's told me on more than one occasion that she wants to hear my release as much as feel it... which of course makes it more intense for both of us."

Lesson for us guys: It's fine, even great to vocalize during sex, but verbalize, too.

7

MATRIARCHAL MOTIVATION

Being Shaped by Her (1.11.07)

Is it unmanly for a husband to want to be "shaped" by his wife? I don't think so, and I'm not alone in the view. A husband-shaping dynamic is very much involved in the idealized wife-led marriage, coveted by those men who pursue this lifestyle. As a recent posting by a husband on a wife-led relationships board explains:

"What I am doing by allowing myself to submit to her is allowing her to shape me into the man she wants me to be. And that man is not wimpy or weak when dealing with the world, but he is very loving and deferential when dealing with his beloved wife."

As another wife-worshipping husband once wrote (in Lady Misato's husbands' forum): "I am proud to be in touch with others who know the true meaning of being a man is found serving and worshipping the woman he loves... [By doing that] you will toss the male ego burden aside. You will be free to grow in your service to her. To be a real man, her man."

These guys make wife worship sound kind of like a spiritual path, don't they? Not that they pray to their wives (though they may bend a knee to kiss her proffered hand or even her dainty toe), or actually worship her (in an idolatrous sense). But they do view each day as an opportunity to perfect their service and devotion to her, to make her the center of their life, the focus of their thoughts and feelings. And in this "centering" they profess to find daily bliss.

Amen to that!

Being Shaped By Her, Part 2 (2.5.10)

The reshaping, or retraining, of the husband/boyfriend is foundational to the female-led lifestyle, whether the regimen is self-imposed by the man or at the behest of the woman.

But hubby makeovers, whether mild or extreme, are part of most marriages, not just the wife-led variety. What bride doesn't envision at least tinkering with the big lug she's hitched to her wagon? Which bride hasn't a list of guy things that need fixing (or nixing altogether) post-nupt?

After all, most guys need whipping into shape by women, since we come clueless, by and large, first into the state of matrimony, then into father- and family-hood. We are clueless, too (if I may generalize), about social etiquette and other refinements of civilized society outside of tailgating and guy-talk.

This renders most males, as far as eligible females are concerned, as works in progress, or fixer-upper houses with possibilities but plenty of problems.

So "Changing Male Behavior," as discussed in other posts, is not just one feature of the female-led relationship. It is at the very core, written into the founding documents, either figuratively or literally. The process may be incremental and insidious, or dramatic and sudden. But it will take place.

"Females are taught by society that it is not right to want to change the male, and that even if it were ethical, it can't be done anyway." one such wife wrote. "This is a lie, foisted upon females by our prevailing patriarchal society. Male behavior will change and improve dramatically when the woman…"

When the woman does what exactly? Well, we'll get to what a woman might do to facilitate those little improvements in a moment. But first let's look at all this female tinkering under hubby's hood from the staunchly male point of view. Typically, or stereotypically, guys are supposed to resent this kind of female meddling with their personalities, or habits, or behaviors, or quirks, or taste in casual clothes, or favorite adolescent breakfast cereal. And many guys do resent this female litany of their shortcomings, and fight it tooth and nail, while giving ground, inch by inch and mile by mile, like a vanquished army in slow retreat.

But men in wife-led marriages, or working toward that blissful state, do not resist the invasive or pervasive influence of their wives, or at least try not to resist. They have decided to let the reshaping process proceed—according to her design and her timetable.

Maybe more husbands should adopt this point of view. Here's a cautionary tale, told me by a middle-aged Latina about her own father, who resisted for decades his wife's attempts to make him go to Mass with the family.

This devout lady got an inoperable cancer in her late '40s and was suddenly taken from him and her children. After burying his wife, the woman told me, her father never once missed Sunday Mass. It is there, in church, praying and taking Communion, that he feels her presence most near.

A touching story. And the moral, I would say, is don't wait for it to be too late to do the right thing. Or, even more specific, to do what your wife asks or pleads with you to do. Do what she says now!

The reshaping process works, as Napoleon Hill commented (in his book *Think and Grow Rich*, and it works for self-improvement like no other incentive. Women have the "power which has done more to help men achieve success than all other forces combined."

In Chapter 7 of my book, "Bonus Points: Motivational Magic," I quote husbands and wives on the success of these wife-inspired marital makeovers—guys losing weight, stopping smoking, getting fit, getting promotions, sometimes with positive, sometimes with negative incentives (yes, punishment can be involved).

Nowadays you can find FLR blogs where hubby's progress is documented, where Coach Wife is helping him get to goal weight, kick a nasty habit (smoking, net porn, "wanking in the loo," etc.).

There are wives who up the ante on their hubby-training in various ways (far beyond the purview of this blog), and husbands who willingly submit to these intense regimens. Think Rocky Balboa, out doing his predawn roadwork, with Adrian driving alongside, shouting in a megaphone.

As one wife comments, "Modifying his behavior can take months or even years of loving manipulation, but it is SO worth it!"

A deeper level of male behavior modification is espoused on the DreamLover Laboratories site, a process they call "Identity Reframing." The idea, explained elsewhere in these pages, is to "get the man to feel pride, rather than shame, in serving his wife, in private or public."

As the author, Kathrin Cohen, explains it: "No male expects you to deliberately try to change his self image. After all, all his subsequent actions will be self-directed and require no intervention from you. He will never suspect that you have been 'customizing' the mental mechanisms that are making all the decisions for him."

If this smacks somewhat of getting Rover to roll over, you're getting the message. On many female-authored FLR websites you will see links to various books and articles on how animal training techniques can be successfully employed on husbands and boyfriends. You'll find no-nonsense titles like these:

How to Make Your Man Behave in 21 Days or Less Using the Secrets of Professional Dog Trainers (by Karen Salmansohn)
The Boyfriend Training Kit (by Tanya Sassoon)
Husband-ry 101, How to Train Your Husband to Be the Spouse You've Always Wanted Him to Be (by Michael H. McCann)
Don't Shoot the Dog!: The New Art of Teaching and Training (by Karen Pryor)
The New Bride's Guide to Training Her Husband (by Emily and Ken Addison)
What Shamu Taught Me About Life, Love, and Marriage: Lessons for People from Animals and Their Trainers (by Amy Sutherland)

The sagacious Fumika Misato goes into considerable depth on behavioral or operant conditioning of the male on her pioneering website, "Real Women Don't Do Housework."

Does this sort of wife-administered Pavlovian regimen work? Apparently so, at least according to this guy: "It is strange that, while I don't really want the various kinds of punishment my wife delivers, at the same time I can't think of a better feedback mechanism to improve my general behavior and performance of my duties."

Being Shaped By Her, Part 3 (2.19.10)

According to Goddess V (from the "Wife-Led Marriage" blog), "There are few limits to how far a dominant wife can push and control her husband if she handles him properly."

Fumika Misato (of "Real Women Don't Do Housework") puts it this way: "You should be able to train your husband to do virtually anything you want."

I am convinced of this. But, if you want additional verification, let me quote a husband from Lady Misato's website: "My wife has been experimenting with the techniques on your website. One thing that concerns me is that there seems no limit to her power over me."

Is his a genuine "concern," do you think, as he feels himself slipping ever deeper under his wife's newfound sovereignty? Or, in the guise of a complaint, is this guy really boasting of his helplessness?

Like this husband, who obviously relishes the way he turns into helpless putty in his wife's capable hands: "At that point, I was so thirsty to submit that I felt there were no limits to my compliance." He adds, in happy hindsight: "An assessment that turned out to be remarkably true."

The point being that husbands, once they have bought into the wife-led concept, seem uniformly to enjoy hands-on training.

"Husbands here seem to fall into two groups," one wag commented on Misato's old Wife Worship Forum, "those who are already being conditioned by their wives, subjected to behavior modification along the lines advocated by Lady Misato, using sex as both the carrot and the stick, and those of us who WISH we were!"

Mistress Kathy, who writes the candid and caring "Femdom 101" blog, likens a husband's enthusiastic response to his wife's commands to the way her uncle's hunting dogs responded to their daily training (and no, she doesn't equate men to canines):

"It was a joy to watch Liz interact with her husband... She worked with her husband almost every day to fine-tune his skills. The smallest finger or hand movement was a signal for him to do something; fetch, come, go, or whatever. Just like my uncle enjoyed working his dogs, she enjoyed working her husband. Just like the dogs enjoyed being worked, her husband enjoyed the feeling of being ordered around and about by his lovely wife."

The application of animal training techniques to husbands and boyfriends, as noted in the previous post, seems to have spawned an Amazon.com book category unto itself, along with a bonanza of magazine and website articles. Some of these articles are quite tame, excuse the pun, with girl-to-girl advice on teaching a guy how to plan a romantic evening—e.g., "Have your favorite chilled wine on hand so you can ask him to open it before dinner." ("6 Ways to Train Your Boyfriend")

Other articles, especially those on female-domination sites, openly advocate rewiring husbands and boyfriends through more invasive means, such as autosuggestion, hypnosis, electroshock, neuolinguistic programming, operant and Pavlovian conditioning, even—say it isn't so!—the prolonged chanting of matriarchal mantras.

Female-empowerment psychologist Elise Sutton takes a more traditional approach in her carefully crafted sequence of "Psychoanalysis of the Submissive Male" procedures. Sutton describes these as "a series of psychoanalysis exercises and procedures to help the dominant woman explore and better understand her submissive man.... [and] to better equip her in taking her proper place in her relationship."

Ms. Sutton's intent, clearly, is to empower the wife as the dominant marital partner, while encouraging the husband to dredge up and focus all his submissive feelings upon his wife. To facilitate the process of psychological surrender, the husband is usually to be naked during Ms. Sutton's procedures, while being interrogated, stimulated and often physically manipulated by his seductively clothed wife.

Hey, guys, like to schedule an appointment?

An even more direct approach to masculine mind control was advocated back in the '90s by a dominant wife called "Madame Rebecca" who operated her own Yahoo! Group entitled, I recall, "Trained Husbands and Happy Wives."

She simply advises husbands: "Let your wife do your thinking." If this seems a bit vague, she spells it out:

"Too many males try to think for themselves. You must learn to allow your Lady to think for you, tell you what to do, what you like, what you are, what you are to think about and such.

You have no need for your own thinking and it will only serve to cause you trouble."

She gets even more specific: "Relinquish all thought process to her and accept whatever she tells you. Don't think for yourself, your lady will do your thinking for you, accept her thinking as your own."

Does that sound, oh, I don't know, a wee bit autocratic? Even dictatorial? But looked at the other way around, from the viewpoint of a husband eagerly seeking to increase his submissive service to his wife, Madame Rebecca is really offering a stirring motivational message. To wit:

"You want her to be more active and you desire to show her you are a useful male and serve her. Does it not appear to you that if she told you or asked you or that if you even thought she wanted you to do something, you should do it? Live for her and let her do your thinking for you. Let her know that you know she is always right and she is smarter than you and knows what's best for you."

I am not advocating this kind of radical female-led mind control, simply including it in the discussion of "being shaped by her." It does exist, and has no shortage of practitioners and proponents. Indeed, many husbands, who initially balk at having their wives mold their thoughts and opinions, become accustomed, and even addicted to the process over time.

Or else!

Like this guy explains: "My wife these days is much less tolerant of my opinion. I can usually only get one of two statements in before she dismisses it. I don't think she realizes the change."

An aspect of female-led thinking that I find particularly interesting, and that some readers will doubtless find controversial (or even shocking), is where a wife imposes her political views on her husband, not only in household discussions but all the way to the polling place.

Judging from many snippets I've collected, it's definitely a trend. Maybe we can chalk it up to feminist payback for all those years of "the little woman" being required to say, "Yes, Dear" to her husband's now-hear-this pronouncements.

Here are some "Yes, Dear" election stories, starting with a husband who identifies himself tellingly as "Mr. Karen": "My wife and I have a system where we vote for only women. If there are no women running for a particular office, we don't vote for it at all. She told me that that doesn't discount the ballot."

Another husband confides to Elise Sutton: "[My wife] has melted her politically radical feminist views (specifically that women should be in positions of political authority) into the fabric of our relationship... we now surf the Internet for sites like 'Emily's List' and 'Wish List' to find female political candidates that we like and we send them small campaign contributions."

Georgeann Cross, in her online book, *Sexual Power for Women*, mentions how, during her senior year at college, she targeted a "short-haired conservative" classmate who got himself elected to the student senate: " I decided I was going to enslave him and make the necessary repairs. If I couldn't change his views, I would at least take control of his vote in the student senate."

Mistress Kathy is equally up front about disenfranchising her submissive husband, or, shall we say, appropriating his franchise: "John is not only allowed to vote, but is required to vote. He, of course, votes the way he is told... This morning John and I went to vote. We voted early. On the way out I asked John who he voted for. He answered 'the way you instructed me to vote, Mistress.' That earned him a 'good boy.'"

Such husbands, you might assume, are surrendering their proxies over to liberal candidates, and you might be right. But not necessarily. As Mistress Kathy goes on to explain, contrasting herself to a dome-wife friend: "While I love [my friend] Liz to death, we are very different people. She is liberal and votes Democratic. I am conservative, and tend to vote Republican. What we have in common is that our guys vote the way we tell them."

The wife-led polling process can be highly erotic, as this wife tells Elise Sutton: "[As election day approached] I had my husband kneel between the couch and the coffee table in our living room and I brought him the checkbook, stamps, envelopes, and information from all the female candidates' websites, complete with a picture of her and address for sending her money... I made him write a check for each candidate (which I signed of course) and prepare all the envelopes to be sent out. I sat behind him on the couch supervising him and gave him an occasional gentle caress. Seeing my scantily clad foot soldier for the female gender on his knees licking stamps and filling out checks and envelopes was very sensual for me and when he was done, I wound up having him bring my vibrator and orally worship me for nearly an hour. I had some of the best orgasms of my life!

"Afterward I did take off his CB and laid him down on the couch and stroked his penis. While doing this, I softly asked him which candidates he found attractive or powerful and I showed him pictures of the ones he identified. I then shifted my focus by telling him in a variety of ways how weak it must make him feel to know that women are taking over society and that his own wife keeps his little cock in a cage and almost totally denied. While doing this I looked into his eyes and saw him in the deepest state of subspace I've ever seen, and he ultimately had by far the most explosive and continuing orgasm I've ever seen him have."

This object lesson in wifely dominion earns an accolade from Elise Sutton (who seems to favor a Libertarian position on many issues): "I think it is wonderful how you used the ever-increasing candidacy of women for high political office to take your husband deeper into submission to you and the female gender as a whole."

Let me add testimonials from two more wife-led husbands, both valued online friends of mine, as it happens, and both utterly devoted to their wives.

Husband No. 1: "my Wife does guide me in all things, including voting. It is only natural as She keeps on top of these things while i tend to the domestic side of life. She reads the front page while i go for the section of the paper dealing with home life."

Husband No. 2: "i am [another] one of the ones whose Wife instructs on how to vote. i was interested in politics and my Wife and i mostly agreed. When we entered on our FLR, my Wife's opinions took precedence and i deferred to Her more and more. i now adopt Her political and business opinions and follow Her lead. She now overrules me when we differ... i just let my Wife make those decisions and i vote the way she tells me. In voting, my Wife will make out a sample ballot or write down who and what to vote for. Occasionally we talk about it, but Her decisions are final."

But at least one female supremacist demurs at this kind of unlimited spousal influence, Katherine West who posts intermittently at "Loving Female Authority": "There is no question," she writes, "that my husband would cast his vote however I tell him, but I also have no desire to rob him of this right."

Such gallant female courtesy to the weaker sex definitely merits an accolade as well, but perhaps not the very last word in this long post. That goes to another anonymous take-charge woman:

"Let's face it ladies, it's quite fun to be in control of a grown male human animal."

Comments:

Runpb: I recently found myself home in the kitchen while my wife went out to vote for president. I was not eligible to vote. (We are citizens of different countries.) She did, of course, cast her vote for the amazing Yulia Tymoshenko of Ukraine. If I had been eligible to vote, there is no question that I would have been influenced to vote in a way in which my vote complimented my wife's vote.

Mknight: Katherine West correctly describes voting as a right but it is also a responsibility and to blindly vote for a woman based on her sex on issues that can effect many other people is dodging that responsibility.

Leslie: I also regard complete female control with skepticism. It is still possible to have a happy, harmonious FLR while allowing the man to retain his individuality and (most) personal freedoms. Just my $.02.

8

BLESSED ARE THE MEEK

Worshipping Your Wife -- Literally? Part 1 (5.8.08)

The short answer is, "Of course not." But, because long-winded answers are my stock in trade, I'm going to unpack "Of course not" into a whole slew of paragraphs, maybe even stretch it out over several posts.

But why even raise the question, you may wonder? Does anyone advocate, or actually practice, idolatry of the female?

Yes, in fact. As I wrote in a sidebar on my wife-worsshsip website (a sidebar not incorporated into the actual book):

"In some female-supremacist organizations, males literally worship females; and in coupled relationships, literally worship their partners (by whatever agreed-upon exalted title). In some instances, there are even religious trappings—thrones and altars and confessions and so forth."

Here's an example, from a letter to Elise Sutton by the daughter of a self-proclaimed goddess: "My Mother was a staunch Female Supremacist. It was her lifestyle and her religion... [My father] had to worship her as his earthly Goddess and be her slave. My Mother had ceremonies and rituals where the men had to worship the women."

"My wife makes me worship her, pray to her and chant to her," writes another husband. "It is a beautiful thing. I humble myself before my wife and pray to her. Then I kiss her feet and slowly work my worshipful kisses up her legs and eventually make my way..."

Heavens! Our devoted husband gets graphically intimate at this point, so let's take an elliptical break... and pick up with: "It is not uncommon for both me and my wife to have tears in our eyes during this sacred ritual."

Another such husband, similarly driven, once asked Elise Sutton: "Is it normal for me to create an elaborate altar that idolizes beautiful women?.. It is about serving a living deity to me."

I like Ms. Sutton's answer: "Women are worthy to be worshipped but you must be careful to worship women in a manner that will meet their practical needs... You can build an altar in your home and meditate all day long but unless you get our there and serve women in practical ways, your faith will be without works and thus be meaningless (to borrow from the Bible)."

She went on to chastise him lightly for his idolatrous theology: "I think you are confusing religion with spirituality. A woman is not a deity nor God. Don't confuse the Creator with the creation."

As I wrote in my online sidebar: "This is not what Worshipping Your Wife advocates. It is not about literal worship (goddess or otherwise), idolatry or anything even remotely sacrilegious. It is about respecting and honoring, revering and protecting, adoring and cherishing."

So, summing up, of course not! I'm not advocating literal wife worship.

Comments:

Enoch: I certainly don't view my wife as a goddess, but I have considered her in a way as a "savior" in that she has helped me to overcome a destructive hobby. The way I see it, she has saved me from wasting my life and freed me from the shackles and chains with which I often saw myself tied to an old hobby.

I also consider her to be Christ-like in that she has forgiven me the enormous pain that my former indifference caused her over many years. That kind of forgiveness is incredible. Given all that, I know she is a person, like me, not a deity or a goddess or a force of nature. I know she has weaknesses, just like I do, and that she needs me to be strong for her just as I need her strength. I view her as my leader, not as my God.

Susan's Pet: I don't try to get religious about my wife or women in general, but I have no problem worshipping one as an earthly goddess. [But] I try not to lose the perspective. One can easily turn fetish itself into the objective, and miss the object of the fetish in turn.

Mark: I like the way you frame it, not getting carried away, but putting your heart into it.

Worshipping Your Wife – If Not Literally, How? Part 2
(5.9.08)

Picking up from the previous post, why do I use the term "Wife Worship" if it's not to be taken literally or seriously?

To quote R.M. Nixon, "Let me say this about that."

Many of us husbands in FLRs do experience strong emotions of reverence and devotion toward our wives. These emotions can be downright intoxicating.

We may even attribute mystical or religious significance to these experiences, seeing our wives transfigured before our eyes as goddesses, or incarnations of feminine perfection.

We intend no sacrilege; I think we just get carried away.

Female supremacists, like Elise Sutton, sometimes refer to these visionary and worshipful states as "sub-space." "Sub" meaning "submissive," which conjures the attitudes and postures of worship, in this case of one's beloved.

However labeled, this amorous intoxication, like any mystical state, is not easily sustained. Nor is it easily forgotten. The afterglow endures and continues to entice.

So a husband inquires on an FLR message board, "Does anyone else out there have a wife-worship mantra running through his head?" Clearly, this is guy is trying to induce his favorite trance-state.

"I've never been able to relate to an abstract concept of God," writes another husband. "Now all my spiritual yearnings have found a focus in my wonderful wife. At times when we are together, I feel the presence of divinity."

What ought a husband to do with these worshipful yearnings? What ultimate purpose do they serve, other than as expressions of devotion?

One might ask the same sort of question of anyone who pursues higher consciousness or any mystical state as an end in itself. What's the point of "illumination" if it doesn't lead to some kind of benign transformation of the one supposedly illuminated?

Let me quote Elise Sutton further on this point: "Meditating before an altar may allow you to show your love, devotion and respect to a deity you cannot see nor touch. But women are amongst you, so in order to love, adore, respect and revere women it takes interacting with them. Women have needs that must be attended to, and I believe man was put here on this earth to meet those needs."

Most devoted husbands have figured this out: "We men aren't learning to serve some abstract entity called 'Woman,'" one man counsels his fellows. "We are learning how to serve specific women, each of whom has highly individualized expectations and desires."

By connecting all the dots in this way, Wife Worship can become a unifying principle and give shape and purpose to a man's life.

"Men were given a wonderful power, a great gift from Mother Nature," writes another man-fan of femininity. "We are capable of tremendous service and sacrifice, when we are truly committed to a goal. We are most content when we have a great adventure before us. We have that cause at the feet of our Goddesses. To lift Them to their rightful roles as the Divine Inspiration to our otherwise sad and empty lives. To give our bodies, our minds, and our lives, to serve and defend these Brave, Beautiful, Nurturing, Challenging, Life-giving, Playful, Wondrous Women. With Their guidance, our lives once again become real and connected to the natural world."

Female supremacist Paige Harrison proudly affirms all these wifely roles in her own marriage: "I am [my husband's] Mentor, Teacher, Priestess, Goddess Queen and the Matriarch of the Family."

To be more explicit, wife worship can be a portal through which a husband is led into a deeper and wider worship, with the wife as his spiritual leader. One wife puts it thus:

"For families that are matriarchal, religion can be made more important and the man can submit to God and his wife so that he can experience the grace he was missing."

"My household is a definite matriarchy and it's Christian," a husband boasts. This man adds that his marital problems were resolved and his faith restored after a female evangelic minister ("Pastor Florence") gave him and his wife a special prayer for daily use. The prayer goes, in part:

"Dear Jesus, let me recognize your image in my wife, and give my wife grace and courage to take the reins of leadership as mother and wife. Help her to lead our marriage with compassion and wisdom. Open my heart to loving submission to You and to her and by this may we avoid a broken marriage and through You may she strengthen my resolve for You."

"My gift of loving submission to her has made my wife blossom into the leader God intended her to be," this husband concludes, "and things are great at church, in our social life, at home, and in the bedroom."

It is even so in my own marriage, I hasten to confess. Like Enoch (commenting on the previous post), my wife has rescued me from wasting my life. I have prospered under her guidance and leadership from the moment I became attached to her romantically.

I have only a few more thoughts on wife-worship and religion, but I'll save them for another post.

Comments:

Enoch: I've seen other men describe being in "sub-space" but have never experienced this myself. However, last night, I had an experience that I thought came close.

My wife was asleep on the couch. We'd had a busy Mother's Day, which included going to a baseball game and having Chinese for dinner. I was still up, as I'd been doing some of the bills on the computer, and I went over to wake her up for bed. She was asleep in a sitting position, and I knelt before her (which I often do), and wrapped my arms around her. And before I tried to wake her up, I just looked at her.

I looked at this wonderful woman and I thought about just how lucky I am. And I could feel the love I have for her welling up inside me as I gazed at her face. And the longer I was like this, the more entranced I felt. She was so beautiful and I was so fortunate.

And as I knelt before her, I thought briefly about your blog-post, about the description of "sub-space" and about the whole idea of wife-worship which you've been talking about in these last two posts.

But mostly I thought about her.

Mark: Enoch, your post reminded me of a like-minded experience once cited on Lady Misato's website— a husband watching his wife as she slept and being overcome by upwelling emotions, culminating in a desire to pay homage to her as a goddess. As I recall, this guy had been a real crummy husband until this "conversion" experience.

Enoch: I just remembered an old episode of "Dallas," where J.R. Ewing had that same reaction. He was gazing down at Sue Ellen, passed-out drunk after discovering he was cheating on her yet again, and he said out loud, "What have I done to you, Sue Ellen?"

Of course, being J.R., this little bit of insight had no lasting effects.

Part 3: Wife-Worshippers as Monks or Fakirs? (5.16.08)

I'm going to explore, ever so briefly and lightly, another way of looking at the wife-led marriage, at least for the husband who has dedicated himself to this way of living, who finds himself drawn to it by deep and enduring feelings.

I'm going to suggest that it can be viewed not just as a life-style choice, but as a kind of spiritual path. And it can be lived as such. on a daily basis. Again, I can speak only about husbands, the worshippers. About the "worshipees," those empedestaled wives who are on the receiving end of daily devotions, I do not venture to speak.

I believe there are some obvious parallels between the man pursuing a deeply wife-led marriage and a person who dedicates himself to a certain spiritual discipline or way of life.

In both instances, there may be a daily sacrifice of certain creature comforts and personal prerogatives in favor of a simplified existence focused on service and devotion.

Whether or not vows are sworn, in either case the individual attempts to set aside his own wants and wishes and to submit his will to that of another. And whether the backdrop be sacred or profane, there can be considerable struggle in this setting aside of one's natural inclinations.

The devotee, in either instance, may be required to sacrifice favorite and even cherished things—hobbies and pastimes, appetites and desires, even traditional rights, as well as bad habits and vices—to keep his pledge and further his quest.

Now this is not intended to be a heavy discussion, just some preliminary thoughts that might, perhaps, provoke serious discussion. That being the case, please don't ask me to what spiritual destination the path of Wife Worship might ultimately lead.

You can give it a name, if you like. Illumination or enlightenment, self-realization or self-actualization. Satori or samadhi. Take your pick. Or maybe that old Army tagline, "Be all you can be." If you prefer something with more emotional or religious impact, then fine, call it salvation.

An interesting description of spiritual disciplines was advanced by the Near Eastern mystic, G.I. Gurdjieff, during the first few decades of the 20th century, and popularized by his most famous pupil, the Russian writer, P.D. Ouspensky. (Books by both men remain in print, and there are thousands of people who profess to be following or even continuing their "esoteric Work.")

Gurdjieff divided the various spiritual pathways, or "Ways," in terms of the physical, emotional and mental disciplines required by each. The "First Way," he said, is more about physical discipline, the "Second Way" emphasizes emotional discipline, while the "Third Way" is all about mental or intellectual discipline. Perhaps "concentration" would be a better word.

In Gurdjieff's shorthand, the First, Second and Third Ways were referred to as the Way of the Fakir, the Way of the Monk and the Way of the Yogi.

The Fakir struggles against the disobedience of the body, forging a sense of will over the physical machine, making it endure pain, etc. (Lying down on a bed of nails, walking on coals, holding one arm aloft for hours, etc.)

The Monk often does likewise, in order to pray without ceasing, ignoring the clamoring of physical and emotional desires in order to focus on God.

The Yogi endeavors to bring body, emotions and mind into a single focus, second by second, minute after minute, in defiance of the entire world of distractions.

Gurdjieff and Ouspensky called their system the "Fourth Way," or the Way of Sly Man. The claim was that the Sly Man must do all these things, and do them while immersed in all the distractions of the world, pursuing the daily business of life. But that is another topic, and preferably for somebody else's blog!

By the way, I make no endorsement of Gurdjieff or Ouspensky: I'm simply borrowing a kind of convenient template for measuring a person involved in a spiritual quest, to see if wife-worshipping husbands might qualify.

And I kinda think they do. As Fakirs sometimes, and Monks, even as Sly Men, secretly pursuing their objectives amid social distractions. Not sure about the Yogi part, though.

Comments:
Enoch: I've been thinking about the terms you present, and yes, like the "Sly Man," I am trying to pursue my objective of submitting myself to my wife, for mutual benefit, amidst all the distractions of daily life—and invisibly to the outside world.

A spiritual path? I dunno... but submission has proven to be a path of self-improvement as I allow my wife to direct me and shape me into the man I was meant to be, instead of the undisciplined boy I was.

Mark: Yes, it's definitely a self-improvement course, if pursued. Daily work on following through on one's aim, unifying one's fractured identity around a central and eminently worthy principle, learning to accept oneself, even those rejected and socially embarrassing aspects, and on and on. With one's beloved as facilitator.

Questioning Manhood (1.14.09)

I cater to my wife. I defer to her judgment, her recommendations, her desires, even her whims, on a daily basis. Most husbands don't act like this, but my contention is that they did, once upon a time. When they were a-courting.

And turning marriage back into passionate courtship is what I both preach and practice.

But, you may ask, is it manly? Or is it wimpish? I ask myself those galling questions more often than you might think. Because I know how I can appear to others. And I have overheard occasional comments from friends or family, male and female, who view me through the optics of traditional masculinity, as less than manly.

Perhaps like the foppish young man in Robert Louis Stevenson's "Story of the Bandbox" (from *New Arabian Nights*), quoted in the very first post of this blog two years ago: "He took a pride in servility to a beautiful woman; received Lady Vandeleur's commands as so many marks of favour; and was pleased to exhibit himself before other men in his character of male lady's-maid and man milliner."

I wouldn't be surprised if, occasionally and safely out of earshot, I am described as tied to my wife's apron strings. Or wrapped around her finger. As spineless, or henpecked. And, to be sure, as pussywhipped.

All true. in a sense. But. arguably. it takes a real man to put up with those kinds of putdowns. Which reminds me of the consoling words of a favorite wife-worshipping mentor. Au876 (from Lady Misato's original husbands' forum):

"I think it takes a real man to properly serve and worship his wife. As husbands it is our challenge to be the real man our wife wants. No matter what it is she wants. we should devote ourselves to her and strive to serve her in every way possible."

Now that I'm pumping myself up. let me venture a bit farther. I contend that catering to one's wife actually builds character. Let me cite. in solidarity. this articulate husband:

"I look at the process of wife worship as part of my growth process as a person. I see the wife worship process as one means to look at my ego. to think before speaking. For instance. I try not to contradict my wife in public or private anymore. So part of the process for me is letting go of certain ego attachments — a big one being the ridiculous need to always be right. even at her expense. Does anyone else out there find himself looking at wife worship as a means of spiritual or personal growth?"

Well. yes. I certainly do. Some of my deferential behavior may be natural inclination. I admit to certain inborn tendencies like Harry in RLS' story. But much of my daily deference involves struggle. I. too. confess to a tendency to interrupt my wife. a compulsion to always be right. My resolve to worship and follow my wife's lead in all things supplies a unity of purpose to my daily life. even moment by moment. helping me to resist these compulsions and modify my natural behavior in her favor.

Maybe I should make a list of some of the stuff I forgo or give up on a daily basis. and happily so. to be more perfectly and ardently hers.

Comments:
Whatevershesays: I've long ago stopped worrying about if others thought I was manly. I guess it doesn't hurt to be 6' 2". 200. And compared to most of my wife's friends' husbands. I can actually handle a power drill. What really matters is if our wife-led marriage makes my wife happy and our marriage

better. For all the guys and women too who think a wife-led marriage isn't "normal," I'll guess yours (marriage) probably isn't perfect. With divorce rate of 50+%, don't knock a wife-led marriage until you try it!

Mark: Agreed on all counts. I'm fairly confident and comfortable in my guy-ness, and equally comfortable with being led by my wife. But I do find myself self-tasked with resolving these disparate selfhoods to my, and my wife's satisfaction.

Jboy: There is great beauty in expressing overwhelming love and adoration for a Woman, in deferring, catering and bowing to her… Your idea of wife worship as character building and as a way for a husband to build himself by letting her mold him into a worthy helpmate is inspiring.

Peace and Contentment (12.18.08)

The other day, while paging through my archives of wife-worship postings, I found an exact phrase cropping up again and again. The phrase was "peace and contentment," and in every instance it was applied to the masculine side of the romantic equation.

Lucky husbands and boyfriends were basically "blissing out," utterly losing themselves in the "Feminine Mystique," over-whelmed and enveloped by goddess-like womanhood.

Here is a short and sweet sampling from men and women alike:

"A wife [may punish] her husband, but afterwards she nurtures him, which brings him peace and contentment." [From Elise Sutton]

"My husband likes being in a constant state of sexual arousal. After I have been sexually satisfied from his body worship and oral servitude, he will lay next to me, exhausted but with the most incredible look of peace and contentment on his face. He is like a helpless puppy dog around me."

"When a man totally surrenders to his wife, he experiences a sense of peace and contentment that he's never known before. I know because I have experienced it."

"I can sense and see the anger and frustration leaving my husband's body when I physically take charge of him, and I see the look of peace and contentment on his face when I am done."

"Let your wife know that you enjoy her power and the more she exercises it, the more it yields the fruit of peace and contentment for you."

"I have been transformed into a happy househusband who has found total peace and contentment in my servitude to my Queen. I never thought I could be this happy and often wonder what took me so long get on the right page."

"When my husband bows before me and worships me as his Queen, and vows to obey me in all things, I feel so powerful and he radiates with peace and contentment. Then I take him in my arms and we both become full of passion."

Comments:
Anonymous: These observations and experiences describe exactly why i desire my Wife to lead me.
Mark: I think this is common to all of us worshipful husbands. It is a happiness, a contentment that nothing else can provide short of some religious ecstasy. But it's pretty near that, as well.

The Primal State of Things (5.1.08)

On the old "Spouseclub" message board (a long-defunct online hangout for corporate househusbands), a member who signed himself "Mr. Louise" spoke frankly, and proudly, of the "blessings" of living in a matriarchy:

"My wife is the absolute center of our home. I have learned complete submission of our finances (though I work, I get an allowance), our home (which means my wife decides all with my loving help, and gives me maternal discipline), and our sex life (which means she decides when, where, and how, which for me as for all submissive men is a thrill). This has led to the blessings of matriarchy: greater harmony, peace, and togetherness... Any one of our friends knows just what I mean when I jokingly say I am under her skirt and that our marriage is a petticoat government. They can see her obvious maternal/matriarchal control over our house and accept us. It is no secret."

In my book I use terms like "wife-worship marriage" or "courtship marriage" instead of "matriarchal marriage" or "matriarchy." Likewise, I advocate a man "court" his wife, "pamper," "adore" and "respect" her, even "defer" to her, rather than, say, "submit" to her.

But in the final chapter, "Happy-Ever-Aftering Takes Work," you will find a fess-up: "If this sounds like modern matriarchy, so be it. According to many husbands who live this lifestyle on a daily basis, it can also be likened to heaven on earth."

Ideally, I should stop relying on euphemisms and drag some of these forthright terms out of the linguistic closet. After all, a WLM, or Wife-Led Marriage, is clearly a matriarchal marriage, in which the husband "agrees" to submit to his wife's authority. And some degree of matriarchy is clearly the governing principle of any FLR, or Female-Led Relationship.

However, I may not be quite ready to embrace that degree of candor, at least in this blog, which, for a number of reasons, I intend to be strongly vanilla-scented and -flavored.

But I will say this. Even the most macho husband, if he truly cherishes his wife, knows that, in a very real sense, he is enfolded and protected by her in the maternal embrace of marriage, just as the developing babe is enfolded and protected in the maternal womb.

"For this cause shall a man leave father and mother, and shall cleave to his wife: and they twain shall be one flesh." (*Matthew*, 19:5, KJV)

So the man is to "leave" one woman only to "cleave" to another, the wife who will replace his mother. Man was obviously not designed to be on his own, however much he may strut about and assert his primacy.

In the wife-led, wife-centered, wife-worshipped marriage, the man fully recognizes this primal state of things and revels in it. To underscore that point, I yield back to that most devoted spouse, "Mr. Louise":

"Now boys, if you will excuse me. I'm going to go and draw Ms. Louise a nice, long hot bath with rosehip and sandalwood oil and fix her tea. She's spent all night at the office and is waiting for my attention. I, as I hope all matriarchal men, would rather wash and massage her body, shave her legs, get her silky robe, spray her aroma therapy, put on her soft music and just listen to her day over chocolate and sparkling wine than almost anything else in God's world."

Letting Him (1.3.09)

I might as well fess up. In my marriage, the impetus for wife worship came from me. I was the one making the sales pitch, though, God knows, it was overdue. I had neglected my beautiful bride in so many ways. In fact, without my "conversion" to this courtship lifestyle, I don't know that my wife and I would still be together.

Her initial skepticism over "wife worship" morphed into a kind of amused tolerance. Of course, I had to prove to her, over time, that this wasn't just another crazy phase. When I began writing the book (intended primarily for her), I think she began to be intrigued.

At one point, when I was outlining all the various topics to be covered, she volunteered to write a chapter of her own: "Letting Him."

I'm still waiting for that chapter, but, in a way, her proposed chapter title says it all. Sure, she seems to be implying, it's male fantasyland, but at least it's putting the husband's focus where it belongs, on the wife. So, ladies, why not let yourself be worshipped as your husband's queen? Or his goddess? Or whatever hyperbolic imagery he prefers.

It's the advice I would give to any wife who is approached by a semi-coherent husband with a tract or printout or webpage advertising the female-led lifestyle or a wife-worship marriage.

Let him—worship you. Serve you. Adore you. Just... let him.

My wife, these days, is doing so. Letting me. Not making a big deal of it. Often not even acknowledging it (best of all). It's routine for me to make our bed, fold her nightgown carefully and lay it under her pillow. To do the laundry, and clean the house, and rub lotion into her lovely feet at night, and be instantly ready for her whenever she initiates intimacy.

And whenever I look around these days, I find another simple service right there in front of me, something to be done for her. A recent example occurred during a holiday trip, where we stayed several days at a hotel.

After we checked in and kind of collapsed, with Christmas packages and luggage all over the place, a lightbulb went off over my head. I remembered a posting on Lady Misato's original Wife Worship husbands' forum from my favorite poster, Au876. I saved it, so I can quote it here:

"We went to visit some of my wife's girlfriends at a lake cabin a couple of years ago. We had to take our own sheets and etc. One of the first things I did after getting the car unloaded was to make up our bed and put our clothes away. Later we were all sitting around talking. My wife asked me, 'Have you made up my bed yet?' One of the ladies started to laugh like that was a stupid thing to expect of a man. But I quickly responded, telling her yes and I had hung up all of her clothes, too...

"The lady who laughed made some sort of comment about what a good husband I was, and my wife responded, saying something like, 'He knows what is expected of him.' I was not embarrassed. I was proud of myself. I had done what I was supposed to do. The fact that my wife asked me was a sure sign she did not intend to keep my devoted status a secret from them. The fact I had already done it was a sure sign to her I was not ashamed of my status."

Flashback to me, with that lightbulb flashing over my head. I was instantly energized. While my wife called our friends in other rooms and made evening plans. I began quietly to unpack, starting with her bag and her clothes, hanging up some items, putting others on a shelf in an adjoining wardrobe area, putting her book and reading glasses and other items on her bedside, her toiletries in the bathroom, then put away her bags. Did the same for me, even made a start with the kids' stuff.

I had never done this simple service before. (Don't ask me why.) But my wife took it for granted, just as Mrs. Au876 had, as if it were expected of me.

She was practicing what she had never gotten around to preaching in that unwritten chapter. She was "letting me."

Comments:
At All Times: I couldn't agree more. It doesn't have to be much more, and what harm is it to let the man who loves and worships the ground that you walk on, express it in a way that could give you both so much pleasure, if only you would let it"

Mark: In a way, "Letting Her" is contrary to the fairly rigid dictum of the "Around Her Finger" Addisons that stealth submission is unworkable, that no progress can be made unless and until the wife asserts her primacy in the marriage.

That's a great way to go, but it isn't the only way. A consistent and incremental and even insidious program of stealth submission by the husband can lead to the wife getting used to being treated as a queen and "letting him" continue to do so. It is, profoundly, a return to courtship. And this second courtship, like the first, has the goal of having the courtee—i.e., the wife—fall in love all over again with the courter. Only it's a different guy than the couch potato guy who takes her for granted.

Anonymous: My father-in-law was the most enslaved, emasculated, hard working, intelligent, submissive man I've ever seen. He was married to domineering "mommy dearest" type wife who could not stand any man except one she could overpower. He is dead now and when she speaks of missing him it is always in terms of what he could be doing for her.

Sean: Re Anonymous' comments regarding his father-in-law. I just want to interject one point: submissive does not mean doormat. While I certainly can appreciate there are men comfortable in completely submissive roles within their marriages, not all FLRs are so one-sided. My wife and I make most decisions together, she values my opinion and while the ultimate decision in matters is hers, very rarely does she completely overrule me. I would also mention that not all FLRs equate to the man doing all the housework. In most households with two working parents, that simply can't work.

Mark: I don't always raise my disagreements with posters, but I agree with you that submissive does not equate to doormat. Our marriage also is two working parents, and most weeknights we're both going as fast as we can just to cover the necessaries—homework, house tidied, kids' messes shoveled aside, dog walked, dinner served, dishes done. Isn't it romantic? And, like your wife, mine does solicit and value my opinion. And then she decides. I don't argue, and don't second guess. She has the right to decide and be wrong. But, doggone it, she's usually right.

9

SURRENDER TO HER GENDER

Enter the Queen (6.2.08)

My wife and I have a favorite line from the movie. *My Big Fat Greek Wedding*. It's the one where the mother. Maria Portokalos (played by Lainie Kazan). tells daughter Toula on the night before her wedding. "The man may be the head of the family. but the wife is the neck. And she can turn him any way she wants."

This always gets a laugh—and. no doubt. resonates as "That's so true!" with most audiences. Haven't we all known for years that wives really run marriages and families? That they just allow husbands. because of their fragile male egos (like Michael Constantine's as Papa Gus in the movie). to pretend to be calling the shots?

But that traditional masquerade is less and less seen in female-led relationships and wife-led marriages. More and more of these wives are dropping the power-behind-the-throne game and openly assuming command. They are issuing edicts in their own names and having their male consorts stand beside. or a little behind. the throne chair now reserved for the Queen.

It's about time. don't you think?

I have been among those wife-led husbands who dream about acknowledging my wife's primacy in public. As if that were some far-off goal on the long FLR road ahead. But if I stop and

155

tote up all the ways in which it is already true, it's obvious that the *fait* is actually *accompli.*

My wife is the head and neck, commanding the orb and scepter of power. Openly so. A few examples should make the case:

1) She pays all the bills when we got out. At restaurants (from fast-food on up), she consults with the kids and me, but has final say on what we can order, from the standpoint of cost, portion-size and what's good for us. It's gotten so that I hardly glance at servers, and they instantly adjust to focus all their attention on my wife. I suspect it's a pattern they are seeing more and more often in couples and families.

2) Ditto when we are on the road—go to a motel or hotel or rent a car, or go to any public attraction where we have to pay. I stand around with the kids while Mom makes all arrangements, especially checking in or checking out at motels. In fact, she often goes in alone, or, if we're with her family, most of whom are female, with another woman, while I wait in the car. (By the way, I never complain or second-guess about any arrangement, motel room, restaurant table, etc.)

3) When we bought our house, and when we went through subsequent refinancings, again, she did all the talking and deciding. More often than not, she used "I" rather than "we" in discussions. The house would be exclusively in her name except that our real-estate guy reminded her that ours was a community property state and that the financing would go better with us both on the dotted line. But when negotiations were in progress, I kept silent unless asked.

And yet, I gripe because on many documents she has me sign above her! It's the same when she tells me to sit at the head of the table when we have company (not always, but often). We still play those charades. But I dare not push her on those small symbolic displays. It's up to her.

And I can be patient. Because we have definitely come a long way down the wife-led path. It was not always thus with us. We were, at the outset, very 50-50. The percentages today are, what, 75-25, 80-20, or even more, in her favor? These days my vote is purely ceremonial, like in the House of Lords.

One might wonder. How much more subservient could I be? Do I *want* to be?

But there are ways in which I could certainly enhance my wife's power and prestige. Without pushing her or "topping from the bottom" or wearing one of those "She's the Boss" shirts or aprons favored by many husbands in FLRs.

I could significantly advance the public aspect of our FLR. I think, simply by following this excellent advice from Au876, a devoted husband who showed the way to me and many others:

"In public and around your friends, one of the best ways to 'continue the relationship' is to take the offense. Don't wait for her to tell you what to do. If she has to do that, people see it as her bossing you around. Jump right in and offer to do this or that or just do it. Treat her like she is the most important and most special person in the world (after all, she is) and you *want* to do these things for her. Do them because you are showing *respect* for her and it won't come across as being submissive. Her female friends will be jealous of her. Your wife will glow in that and appreciate the way you behave in front of her or your friends.

"There is a tendency among men to put down their wife in public. The exact opposite should be the case. Anyone who has a wife they can love, adore and worship is lucky. I consider myself extremely lucky."

Feel the Power! (7.2.08)

Some husbands and wives in long-term FLRs report that their daily life feels kind of vanilla, more or less as it was before the power exchange of putting the wife in charge.

But, then, you usually find that the power exchange is always there, a kind of subtle subtext to every conversation. A look, a word, a hint from the wife is all it takes for her to reassert her authority over him, and for his submissive side to snap to attention.

In other cases, the couple may appear vanilla in social settings, yet with the ever-present threat of the wife playfully "outing" the husband's submissiveness, to whatever extent she chooses. A case in point:

"My wife likes to keep our power exchange mostly secret, yet at the same time she loves to tease me by hinting to neighbors and friends about what a 'henpecked' husband I am. This 'henpecking' suits her dominant nature and my submissiveness perfectly. By stretching my limits in this way, she has made our power exchange a reality. There is no turning back for either of us. She is as addicted to her current level of control as I am to my current lack."

In other words, the female-male power exchange is always there, a palpable thing, whether cleverly veiled or revealed in all its glory.

This radical imbalance of power between the female and male is probably the defining quality of an FLR, more than the presence or absence of certain behaviors or rituals. Conversely, a couple can work their way through a daily checklist of D/s practices and be merely going through the motions, without the underlying reality.

This is what sets FLRs, or WLMs (wife-led marriages), apart from the fantasy worlds of femdom. A wife-led marriage is not a make-believe dressup game until the novelty wears off. It is daily reality—at the breakfast table, watching TV, getting the kids to bed, wherever and whenever. Throughout, the wife never loses her mantle of power, her orb and scepter, her crown.

As Lady Misato ("Real Women Don't Do Housework") has written, "Marriage is an institutional vessel within which the power exchange may occur. In effect, it makes the investment worthwhile."

And in a wife-led marriage, or "wifedom" as Lady Misato has called it, no matter how trivial the pursuit or mundane the circumstances. the husband never loses his sense of healthy respect and even awe for who this woman is in his life. The power that flows from her is something he can feel whenever she is near. or speaks to him. whether or not she is even asserting her primacy over him.

As one husband notes. "For years I had read about the power exchange inherent in FLRs. Well. now I know what it means. I no longer look at my beloved bride the way I did. Whenever I think of her. whenever she is in the room or speaks. there is an aura of power that surrounds her. And. yes. it is sexy. And she knows it. too."

Again. this is not some fantasy that an addle-pated husband superimposes over his wife to spice up his life. And it's not because the wife is swathed in furs. or sheathed in wet-look vinyl. It's because the husband is seeing her. and valuing her. as she truly is—the goddess by whom. miraculously. he is owned.

He knows. of course. that her word is law. no matter how softly spoken or politely couched.

It is certainly so in my case. As with other wife-led husbands. I know that she controls all the money. and how it is spent. and all our schedules. long-term and short. and what we will do. and what we will eat. and. of course. all our sexual activity. I know that I will and must turn to her for advice on all matters. large and small. because her judgment and practical sense so far exceed my own. And that I will benefit and prosper from her wisdom all the days of my life.

So. yes. my wife has been owed deference and worship and obedience from me all these years. And now. finally. she's getting it—and I'm starting to "get it."

Give It Up to Your Queen! (7.08.08)

There's an oft-quoted bit of conventional wisdom that goes
something like this: "Any relationship is under the control of the
person who cares the least."

Where did I see that first? Ann Landers? Dear Abby? Dr.
Laura? Take your pick. I check Google, and the miraculous engine shows me that psychiatrist Gordon Livingston has a lot to
say about it in his book, *Too Soon Old, Too Late Smart*, and that
the phrase shows up in the lyrics of at least one country-western
song.

By whomever codified, the little truism certainly resonates,
doesn't it? Because too many of us have been there and done
that, or been done that. A romantic relationship can be a very
bumpy ride indeed for the person who cares the most.

So if you're in that position, especially where there's a large
imbalance of power, take your foot off the gas and reach for the
brake pedal instead! At least that's what many relationship psychologists advise, if you want to avoid an emotionally
devastating smashup.

However—

In Female Led Relationships, 50-50 is out the window and
everything is topsy-turvy. Here, where the imbalance of power
could hardly be more extreme, with the wife often in control of
every aspect of the relationship, you find results (based on overwhelming anecdotal evidence) that are rewarding and positive
for both.

The greater the imbalance of power, when you're talking female-led, the greater the romantic and erotic potential... and the
fewer arguments or domestic disputes. Where the wife rules, and
the husband follows, as the epigraph to this book proclaims,
"things go well and love is in the air."

This is why, on the issue of power imbalance in a relationship, the leading lights of the FLR movement all dispense advice
that is totally contrary to that of most psychologists. Wives and
husbands alike are urged to take their feet off the brake pedal

and go full speed ahead.

For instance. Fumika Misato (quoted in Chapter 6 of my book) counsels a new-to-the-lifestyle husband to "Consider a true and honest confession of your feelings to your wife. Express yourself without reservation. Don't be afraid to let your wife know how powerful she is."

Or take Au876. also offering advice to a wife-worship newbie: "It sounds like your wife is on the road to taking charge. I hope you will not resist her or try to hold any power for yourself that she wants. Serve her with a smile!"

FLR couples counselor Paige Harrison explains: "My concept is to help the submissive male understand his role to worship. adore and obey his dominant wife or female partner. Learn how to lower yourself to your knees and worship her."

For those of a certain age. this may recall the *Surrendered Wife* concept of Laura Doyle or the *Total Woman* of Marabel Morgan. both of whom held that the secret to a blissful marriage is for wives to cater to their husbands in the bedroom and out. With the proviso. of course. that FLRs turn that traditional advice upside-down.

"What better life [for a man] is there than to serve a superior lady?" Elise Sutton asks rhetorically. "A man's masculinity is complimented when he humbles himself to serve a woman."

And she proceeds to lecture another husband. who has voiced misgivings about certain aspects of the lifestyle. "Your life should be a life dedicated to serving your beautiful Mistress. After all. she deserves your love. devotion and complete obedience... [It is clear in your letter that] you revel in your wife's power over you."

And the formidable Ms. Sutton positively unloads on another husband with last-minute misgivings about relinquishing marital control: "What is your problem? You know you love submitting to your wife so just relax and get with the program... Why do you have to retain some control? Your wife has it right. Men should submit to women and the husband should submit to his wife... you should count your blessings. Forget your male pride

and humble yourself before your wife. Tell her that you are eager to serve her as often as she desires. Cherish your wife and
serve her like the Queen that she is."

The Addisons, Emily and Ken, of "Around Her Finger" fame,
jointly propose that, during an initial trial phase, wives make a
formal declaration to their husbands of the power imbalance that
is to be a cornerstone of their wife-led relationship:

"As you approach the last night of the trial period, have him
write you another letter telling you his thoughts and feelings
over the last two weeks. On the last night, have him kneel naked
in front of you and read the letter to you.

"At this point you will make a decision regarding whether or
not you want to continue with a wife-led relationship. I suspect
that you will both have enjoyed it tremendously and that neither
of you could imagine abandoning it. Importantly, if you decide
to continue, make it very clear to him that you expect your authority to be respected, and that you expect his continued
obedience."

Might that naked, kneeling husband be having some chills
along with his erotic thrills? Could be. It's risky, handing over
that much power to your wife, deliberately placing yourself in a
classic posture of physical and emotional vulnerability. But
aren't risk and vulnerability part of the thrill of original courtship?

A husband comments on this delicious predicament: "Relinquishing total control to a loving trusted spouse provides a base
thrill. Not the thrill of taking your hands off of the steering
wheel while going 75 mph, but knowing that your life will be
controlled by another, to such detail as decided upon by the
dominant partner."

As I wrote in my book (Chapter 6, "Daring to Be Known by
Her"): "The goal here, of course, is not to hide one's worshipful
feelings from one's beloved, but to reveal them. Don't try to be
the 'strong, silent type' when it comes to your adoration and devotion."

I yield the last word to a longtime professional domina,

Dianna Vesta: "There is no greater sight nor braver man than one who melts to his knees, relinquishing control to the one he adores, doing anything that will please her."

Comments:

Mistress Kiara: "There is no greater sight nor braver man than one who melts to his knees, relinquishing control to the one he adores, doing anything that will please her." How beautiful. I've never heard this until now.

Susan's Pet: This balance-of-power concept is the fantasy of men mostly. But I disagree with a lot of what you claim (unless I misunderstood you). "The greater the imbalance of power, when you're talking female-led, the greater the romantic and erotic potential... and the fewer arguments or domestic disputes. Where the wife rules, and the husband follows, as one such wife put it, "things go well and love is in the air."

That goes true for the bedroom. It fails in everyday life. I can see a balance of maybe 60/40, but not much more. The problem is that in what I call normal relationships, both partners need some satisfaction, regardless of what their needs are. Going deeper than 60/40, one of them is not getting enough. Give him or her time, and the relationship will break.

Mark: SP. The power imbalance that I've encouraged in our marriage is part fantasy, but part reality. I do rely on her judgment over mine. But the satisfaction and pleasure I derive from the FLR is probably more like 60/40 in my favor, though I hope hers will increase.

Growing Into the Role (10.16.08)

An elderly friend told me about this girl he knew years ago in college. A real "glamour-puss" (his old-timey word, not mine) who landed the lead in a school play about Queen Elizabeth I (by Maxwell Anderson, I think). She got so caught up in the regal role, issuing orders to bowing and scraping boy-courtiers, that she started acting like an absolute monarch around campus. My friend remembers almost bumping into her one day, whereupon she thrust out an imperious hand and ordered him: "On your knees, vassal, and kiss my hand!"

My friend was having none of it. But while nodding at what-ever point he was making, I was thinking, why couldn't it have been me she ordered to grovel? I wouldn't have hesitated—not back then, not ever. To the best of my recollection, my female-worshipping syndrome kicked in around the age of 3.

Okay, so why did I bring this up? Not to illustrate the foibles of method acting, overidentifying with a part, but to illustrate that our wives (or girlfriends) can gradually grow into the role of our sexy sovereigns, exercising more and more authority over us while accepting our passionate worship.

But we may have to give them time, and encouragement, to help them get comfortable in the new role, to realize how regal and magnificent they are to us (their knights and courtiers).

Female empowerment psychologist Elise Sutton explained it this way to one devoted husband: "Your wife is still new to this lifestyle and you need to allow her to experiment with her fe-male power so she can become comfortable [with it]. Your position is to encourage her and to support her. Let her know that you enjoy her power."

Fumika Misato is even more emphatic: "Let your wife get comfortable with her new role, and you will be set for life."

In fact, female-led relationship message boards are cram-full of postings by husbands sharing tips and comparing notes on how to encourage and empower their wonderful wives, like these:

"My wife feels a little guilty about being spoiled but stills lets me do it. She sometimes points out things that could be done but doesn't correct me much or complain. Yesterday she came home from shopping with some cleaning items that 'you might want to use' and some menu suggestions."

"Last weekend my wife sent me out shopping for household things, telling me what to get. It was very much like the boss telling you what to do. It was fun. Later I think she felt a little guilty about it."

"My wife is happy to be in control of my orgasms. It may take some time before she will feel comfortable to admit it, but I think she will make this arrangement more explicit in the future."

Another husband says his wife is taking "this female-led thing" at her own pace, working to "de-program herself from many years of conditioning as a traditional, non-assertive wife."

"The key," Elise Sutton instructs another husband, "is for you to be supportive and allow [your wife] the room to grow. Encourage her to be in charge and compliment her often... If she makes a mistake, be quick to forgive and be there to serve. Patience on your part is a must."

How does a husband actively encourage his wife to blossom from commoner into queen? How about just start treating her like royalty? Here, from Chapter 2 ("Making Her Your Fantasy") of my book, is the testimony of a wife on the receiving end of such nonstop adoration: "I'm in my fifties and gravity is winning more and more every day. But in the eyes and mind of my husband, I am beautiful—I am his queen—and he shows it to me every minute of every day."

To paraphrase my favorite epigraph ("If you want our wife to be a goddess, worship her"): "If you want your wife to be a queen, obey her." Remember, as Lady Misato said, once she is convinced of your sincerity and your passion, you'll be set for life.

But what does that mean? What's it like living with an emerging goddess?

"Very interesting" is this husband's initial reaction: "It's been very interesting to see how my wife is slowly changing the more comfortable she gets in the superior role within our relationship, the more she gets comfortable with the idea that she has all this power and sees what effect she has on me."

For this husband, the elevation of his spouse into queenly status means that he is privileged to kneel in her presence, a long-cherished desire of his, as it happened: "I did not beg to kneel before my wife and worship her, but just expressed my feelings about it several times. All I wanted was to be heard, and felt that I should not push her. The sincerity did the trick. She no longer saw it as slavish behavior but as a deep-seated desire of her husband."

The abiding gratitude this guy felt when his worshipful wish was granted is echoed by many husbands in wife-led unions: "Have you ever thought of what a wonderful gift our wives give us by accepting our worship? I pleasured her this a.m. and without a word she just fell asleep when she was done. It makes me feel great to see her relax that much and to know that I've contributed to it by not making demands on her for my pleasure."

The more completely their wives identify with their queenly role, it seems, the happier their husbands: "My Wife/Goddess has gotten very, very comfortable with this lifestyle. After one bad argument, my Queen put her foot down and laid down the law! Today our marriage/life is lived the way SHE wants it to be. Even if I ever had 2nd thoughts and asked to go back to normal, this is something she would not accept. She is too comfy in her view on life as a Goddess and living a female led relationship."

"I have never felt so much love and adoration for my wife. I surrendered our home life to her and it has only gotten better. I don't know when it happened exactly but during the course of releasing control to my wife, I realized that I could trust her with anything. That is a very powerful and wonderful revelation to experience but it is also fundamental, I believe, to a successful female-led marriage."

"My wife is increasingly comfortable with her authority over me," boasts another husband. He goes on to explain how, as he served her the dinner he had just prepared, she proceeded to outline his schedule for the next week and weekend: "'Yes Ma'am,' was all I said, but her tone of voice and her certainty went directly to my heart—and groin. It was slightly embarrassing."

And what of the newly crowned queens? What say they?

Here's a spirited sampling:

"I have entered a whole new world of power. It took a few months for me to get on top of things, but I have him so worked up and attentive, keeping the house in order just the way I like it.

I truly feel and know I am a Goddess now!"

"I love men who really care about. worship. adore. and submit to the will of Women. not caring about their own petty interests and hoping with devout sincerity to please the Lady of their affections. And I am so lucky that my husband is just such a man!"

"I can't imagine any woman not loving to be worshipped by the man she loves. especially seeing him having the guts to do it openly and publicly."

"I just love the power rush!"

"I was always sorta shy. but now I'm confident. assertive and very comfortable with myself. My husband has given me all this and much more. I am in charge of lovemaking - I decide when we do it. how we do it. whether he can penetrate me and whether he can bring himself to a climax. This might sound very controlling. but in fact my husband says it has given him an aroused state of being for hours or even days. And I am certainly enjoying it!"

"The control I have over my man just floors me."

"I'm 23. so maybe it's a generational thing. but I can't imagine any woman not loving this. In fact. the group of women that I hang out with are all determined that we will be in control in our relationships. I think the ideal of equality that women talked about in the sixties and seventies ridiculous. Why should women settle for equality? Why should they settle for anything less than being totally in control?"

"Remember that your husband craves your authority." one wife counsels another. newer to the lifestyle. "Even if you think it sounds like a bit much to say it. tell him that he must obey you. Tell him you are in charge. He wants – he needs – to hear it."

"Embrace your authority." advises Emily Addison on the "Around Her Finger" blogsite. "Throttle this [female-led] dynamic to your comfort level."

End result—"Happy-Ever-Aftering." as I titled the final chapter of my book. But with. perhaps. a cautionary whisper to husbands embarking on this journey from one who's been there and done that: "The biggest danger is opening the Pandora's Box of possibility. A wife acculturated by a lifetime of deference and submission to men may discover an authoritarian role she didn't know she could have, and she might like it. And she may not want to go back to the way things were, even if you suddenly change your mind."

Be prepared, in other words, once you have assisted your wife onto the household throne, to play your supporting role in a long-running play. Not "Queen for a Day" but "Queen for Life."

Comments:

At All Times: I am going through the same phase in my own developing WLM. It has taken me a very long time to reach the same conclusion and realize just how important it is just to let your wife grow into her dominant role and discover for herself how best she can demonstrate and use the feminine power that she has over me. Not only is this better for her, but as a result it feels that much better when things come from her, rather than encouraged by me.

Jason: This is something my Wife has had the hardest time with. Sometimes, as a simple knee-jerk reaction I may talk back or disagree, and she seems to fold immediately. She knows she's in charge on a mental level, but emotionally she never stands up to me, or puts me in my place... It's like she refuses to truly accept her mantle of authority, even though we both know it's there, and we both know she wouldn't want it any other way.

Mark: As that TV commercial says, "I'm so there" with both you guys. Encouraging (and not undermining) my wife's preeminence in our marriage has been, and continues to be, a long march.

At All Times: In order to encourage your wife's increasing control and dominance you have to let your wife see the effect that she is having on you. There is no point in offering to submit to your wife, unless you are prepared to submit fully and let her see by your actions and response that she can control you in the way that she will eventually enjoy herself.

Jboy: I have found that asking your Wife's advice, opinions and direction in many areas is very helpful in building her confidence and lets her see herself in a leadership role. I always ask my Wife's advice (especially since she is so often right) and follow her carefully. Since things usually come out well, I truthfully praise her as the wise one in our family.

Anonymous: I don't dare let my submissive needs be known to my wife not only because I am afraid she might reject them, which I am, but also because I am afraid she might embrace them.

I am afraid that I may not be ready for such a dramatic change in my life-style. Some days I totally want to do it, but I'm a lazy man and my wife is very active. When she pursues a goal, she is relentless, so I fear that her rule, much as I desire it, may be more than I can handle.

Both scenarios are scary to me, so I live in constant frustration.

Her Wish Is My Command (4.1.09)

All teaching, I once read, can be divided into three forms:
1. Example
2. Hint
3. Impetus

The point I recall being made is that "Example" is most effective, "Impetus" least, with "Hint" somewhere in the middle. Teaching by example is pretty obvious; "impetus" equates to direct commands; while "hint" covers just about everything else, from harangues to hypnotic suggestion, lectures, textbooks, maybe even the unimaginable whole of Wikipedia.

All three styles are employed by good classroom teachers, of course; or maybe, in higher educational jargon, they're called "pedagogical modalities."

Of course, all three forms are equally in play in Wife-Led Marriages or Female-Led Relationships. Let's start with "impetus."

Prurient literature of the female supremacist genre used to favor the autocratic Victorian schoolmistress issuing directives, punctuated with well-aimed slaps from a ruler. We're definitely talking "impetus" here.

Judging from the WLM and FLR forums and message boards I've frequented over the years, real matriarchal martinets do exist, but are more likely to be creatures of male fantasy than flesh and blood.

The extreme autocratic wife issuing arbitrary "Now Hear

This!" commands is probably role-playing by mutual consent, with both parties reveling in the delicious topsy-turviness of it all. Full-time, non-stop role reversal tends to be derailed by the little distractions life throws our way, like holding a job and raising kids.

Far more common, and more powerful, I think, are wife-worship or wife-led marriages where the woman leads by "example" and "hint."

How by "example"? Perhaps just by being herself. My wife doesn't have to put on queenly airs to be a queen, in my view. She just *is* one. In fact, she plays her regality down (in terms of the Power Distance Index, as described by Malcolm Gladwell in his best-selling *Outliers*.)

In general, wives are far more likely to employ hints than ultimatums, subtle cues than imperious gestures. The difference in Wife Led Marriages is that husbands learn to pay attention to these cues, to interpret these hints, and eventually to treat them as directives.

"Your wish," the courtier-husband says to his queen-wife, "is my command!" Or perhaps: "Your hint is my impetus!"

A textbook example was supplied in the (now inactive) blog of fdhousehusband:

"In the early days, my Wife would say something like, 'My carpooler went home early so I'll be taking the bus home today.' i just accepted that like She was giving me a bit of information. What She really was saying was 'I need you to pick me up from work.' Once i understood the Female language, i learned to respond by saying things like 'May i pick You up from work today?' i found that She really responded to these 'offers' to do things for Her which She in fact had prompted with subtle 'requests.' i also think that it showed Her that i was really listening to everything She was saying."

According to Fd, he actually taught himself how to decode "female language" by studying books by sociologist Deborah Tannen, especially *You Just Don't Understand: Women and Men in Conversation*.

Fd provides another example (using ultra-feminist spelling and capitalization): "Even with my Wife, i've had to read between the lines. Today, She called me at work to tell me that one of our daughters was at a friend's house and that it was getting late. If a Womyn gives you a piece of irrelevant information, look at it carefully and try to figure out why she would be telling you that. i immediately read it as 'I need you to go pick her up.' So i said to Her, 'I'll leave now and pick Her up on the way home.' She said, 'That would be great Sweetie.' Womyn speak in a different language and that is why such gender language books are so valuable."

Another husband quick-on-the-uptake when it comes to wifely hints was the oft-quoted (by me) Au876. "I seldom if ever ask her what she wants me to do next. I know what she expects and I do it without asking. She often drops gentle hints which I respond to as though they were absolute commands. Our relationship is such that I consider any hint or suggestion by her as a direct order. She is just as likely to say 'Would you like to vacuum the den?' as 'Go vacuum the den.' Either way I go vacuum the den."

As such female-led relationships mature, of course, the wife may grow comfortable with a more direct communication style.

A current WLM blog, "At All Times," offers an example of a wifely progression from indirect to direct:

"Jane's attitude is changing towards what and how she expresses herself towards me... we had been shopping together, and had forgotten several things. Jane called out to me, 'We have forgotten this and that, do you want to go back to the shop?' When I replied, 'Not really' in a less than enthusiastic voice, Jane was quick to add, 'But you're going, aren't you?' Realising my mistake, I said, 'Yes, of course,' and so it was that I had to go back, because Jane had insisted."

Jane's husband clearly could improve his female literacy skills, so that those "But you're going, aren't you?" reminders could become less frequent and things could go as smoothly as for this wife-led couple:

"We believe that she can be totally and really in charge without raising her voice at me (except when I really deserve it) and with her showing as much respect and affection for me as I for her."

Pointed reminders, even schoolmarmish lectures, however, may be required on occasion, in the wife-led home as in the classroom, as this husband learned:

"The most satisfying and exciting part of my marriage is doing what my wife wants. I would not have been able to do that if she had not been willing to assert her wants and to coach me on how to best fulfill them. Men are dense. If my wife's 'asserting' and 'coaching' had come in subtle signals rather than explicit requests, I wouldn't know half as much about her today. We agreed that she did not need to pull her punches to spare my feelings."

If your husband continues to tune you out, this matriarchal Ms. suggests, get in his face: "Sit him down, shut off the TV, get his undivided attention and talk to him until he is dismissed. While you are talking to him, remember that women and men think differently and it is your responsibility to be heard—to teach your [husband] how to hear you. Women like to give subtle hints while men need a flare gun shot at their heads to get the point."

"Flare gun" may be a bit strong. A rolling pin is more traditional--right, Enoch?

Comment:
At All Times: I think Jane's husband knew exactly what he was saying, and as a result got the type of response he was looking for.

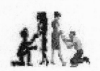

The Power Transfer (4.23.08)

Those involved in "alternate lifestyles" sometimes refer to a "power transfer"—the process of imbalancing or tipping the relationship dynamics in favor of one partner over the other.

In FLRs, or female-led relationships, the transfer is done in favor of the woman. And, since we're clearly talking about consensual relationships, that means the man has voluntarily ceded some of his power or authority over to the woman, to create an imbalance that both partners may find stimulating.

"Right now I am really feeling her power over me."

The quote is from Au876, one of the mainstays of Lady Misato's original husbands' forum on Yahoo. He goes on: "Guess I better go iron her blouse and maybe find some surprise chore to complete that she will notice."

This shows the kind of provocative imbalance that can exist between worshipped wife and worshipping husband, another aspect of the queen-knight paradigm. The queen has merely to enter the room and her knight-courtier is instantly alert to serve her in some way.

But Au876 was quite clear that he had, at some point, given that power to his wife. And just as clear that he liked it that way, and didn't want it back.

"Our relationship just sorta evolved," he explained. "At one time my wife did everything and I did nothing. I am not even sure how it evolved, but today it is almost completely reversed. It really makes me feel good to be, say, fixing her dinner while she is watching TV or napping or reading the paper. The doing of it makes me feel good, and the fact that I am doing it for her makes me feel good."

But why would that be?

Why wouldn't a husband prefer to sit back, watch the Game on TV and have his wife cater to him?

Why not indeed?

Because Au was endlessly courting his wife, day after day. That was the life he lived, and chose to live. The Power Exchange makes little sense without that. With the added element of daily courtship, it makes perfect sense.

The suitor grants the object of his affections power over him, awaits her verdict on his feverish hopes and dreams. He is perfectly transparent to her in his adoration, while she is veiled in regal mystery. While he awaits her verdict, he does everything he can to please her, to cater to her and curry favor.

Courtship is Power Exchange, instilling a kind of giddy daily bliss in certain men, a courtship that never ends.

Power Games (2.2.10)

In the posting "Give It Up to Your Queen!" I cited the trite "truism" that "Any relationship is under the control of the person who cares the least." The idea, apparently, is to guard against being seen as caring too much—especially when you do!

But protecting yourself in the intimate clinches is not a smart tactic in romantic relationships. It can lead to many things, but happily-ever-aftering is probably not among them. Far better, at least according to us wife-worshippers, to open your heart and mind completely to the object of your adoration—"Daring to Be Known by Her," as I titled a chapter of my book.

Withholding from her, or from him (for that matter), how you really feel can lead to the missed opportunity of a lifetime.

A classic example, where both parties realize the price they have paid for their subterfuge, is the final denouement between Rhett and Scarlett in *Gone With the Wind*. Too late Scarlett realizes and blurts out her true feelings to the man she has considered all these years a "ruffian" and a "scoundrel" and—well—"no gentleman."

By the last reel, of course, Rhett no longer gives a damn. The last time he did care, as he tells her, is when he grabbed her—his own wife—and carried her upstairs "into the swirling darkness." to ravish her and. he hoped. entirely expunge the image of Ashley Wilkes from her brain. Then. alas. as he explains (p. 1031 of the Macmillan hardcover):

"I was afraid to face you the next morning. for fear I'd been mistaken and you didn't love me. I was so afraid you'd laugh at me I went off and got drunk. And when I came back. I was shaking in my boots and if you had come even halfway to meet me. had given me some sign. I think I'd have kissed your feet. But you didn't."

Scarlett answers: "Oh. but Rhett. I did want you then but you were so nasty! I did want you! I think—yes. that must have been when I first knew I cared about you... but you were so nasty that I—"

Rhett's classic reply: "It seems we've been at cross purposes. doesn't it?"

Of course. the Rhett-Scarlett Power Game. permuted over all those tumultuous decades. is the engine of the book (and film). and keeps us reading and watching *GWTW* over and over. But the unhappy upshot of the power game persists. even after marriage. when hero and heroine are supposed to live happily ever after.

To avoid such tragic cross purposes. Lady Misato (as quoted in Chapter 6 of my book) counsels the "tell-all" approach to husbands: "Consider a true and honest confession of your feelings to your wife. Express yourself without reservation. Don't be afraid to let your wife know how powerful she is."

The advice is applicable the other way round. as well. Drop the game and let yourself be vulnerable!

There was a book that espoused this idea. many years ago—basically to dote on your spouse. instead of playing power games. Only this advice was directed not to husbands. but to wives. The book. *Surrendered Wives* by Laura Doyle. is still selling briskly. with ancillary audio cassettes and seminars. (Actually Doyle's book echoes many of the prescriptions of an earlier anti-feminist best-seller. Marabel Morgan's *The Total*

Woman.*)

(* "Mr. Lynda," who relished being under the thumb of his take-charge wife, "Ms. Lynda," on the old Spousechat message board, apparently followed some of Marabel Morgan's more playful prescriptions—in reverse: "I found a book entitled *Total Woman* that was written in the late sixties or early seventies by a woman who told other women how to keep the home fires burning... I have done some of those things in reverse. Have you ever stripped for Lisa, and been her naked servant for the evening?")

I recall the "Surrendered Wife" idea being bandied about on Lady Misato's original husbands' forum, one member dismissing it as "Stepford Wives' tales."

Another guy opined: "Effectively, it's Wife Worship in reverse! Now, this poses some very interesting questions: Is the key to a perfect marriage that one partner submits to the other, not really mattering which one submits to which? Is Lady Misato wrong and whoever it was wrote *Surrendered Wives* right, or vice versa? Or are they both right and wrong at the same time? I'm not sure I have all the answers, but doesn't being a 'surrendered wife' simply mean that you are doing what your grandmother or even your mother did before you, except they did not have a choice and you do? Boring, ain't it?"

Another commented: "I do not feel comfortable with your postulation that wife worship is merely Surrendered Wives in reverse. Men are bigger and more aggressive. A woman's control rests on moral ascendancy. Let me postulate it as a step forward in the evolution of human society and pronounce Surrendered Wives an atavism."

Lady Misato settled the debate: "Let me pipe in here with one philosophical point: Marriage works better when one partner submits to the other. I happen to believe that it is more interesting, effective and, indeed, natural for the husband to submit to the wife. I have not read the book (I ought to) but I suspect most if not all of the reasons cited are entirely valid, only I doubt there is any strong reason in support of the husband being the head.

Remember, [in a wife-worship marriage] you are not abrogating responsibility, only submitting your will to hers. She'll load you with your responsibilities."

Let me offer the parting shot on this topic to Mistress Kathy of the "Femdom 101" blog:

"No matter what the experts say, marriage is simply not 50 50: somebody has to ultimately [have] the last say. Women tend to dominate men even in so called vanilla marriages with no overt D s. Why not simply bring it out into the open and once and for all settle the matter and concede that the wife should be boss?... I mean what is the big deal about it?"

Comments:

Runpb: Growing up, my father was very authoritarian. His word was law... with the kids and with my mother. (It wasn't until the last few years that my mother was allowed to wear pants outside the home!) I could always tell that she wanted needed more room to breath.... to relax... to be herself. Today both my parents quietly observe my wife and me. I am openly submissive to her. We both are comfortable and happy in our roles. Oddly, my father adores her and my mother seems a bit jealous or suspicious or her. We are clearly more happy in our marital relations than they ever were.

Anonymous: The whole Surrendered Wives thing seems like an attempt to resurrect "Leave It To Beaver." If some women (or a lot, in this case) are into the submissive role, that's certainly their prerogative. I'd wager that a "Surrendered Husbands" version wouldn't go down quite so well, though.

Mark: runpb & anonymous, glad to see that you're both onboard with the idea of surrendered husbands. Granted, it would be a stretch to envision Rhett Butler fetching for and doting on Scarlett, but then again, he does talk about kissing her feet, and that would certainly make for a more provocative GWTW sequel than has been offered so far by Alexandra Ripley and Donald McCaig.

She Decides, I Abide (5.30.08)

My parents argued an awful lot. Even when they weren't arguing, there was too often a palpable air of cold hostility around the house.

Not fun.

My wife and I never argue. Well, almost never. Nor are we, I venture to boast, storing up grievances and recriminations for later use—like maybe in divorce court.

What's the secret?

As I wrote in my book's final chapter, "Happy-Ever-Aftering Takes Work":

"At some point... I stopped arguing with my wife. Not all at once, and not without occasional blowups or fits of masculine pique, but gradually I began accepting what we had both known for years—that things work out better when we do them her way."

Here's how another husband puts it: "I no longer mind that she is so often right. I can deal with it—happily, in fact."

And another: "I have found that not bickering is a refreshing way to live. It's about deferring to her."

And finally: "We get along really well because there is no power struggle."

It's even scriptural, according to St. Paul's injunction (1 *Cor.* 1:10): "Now I beseech you, brethren, by the name of Our Lord Jesus Christ, that you all say the same thing; and there be no dissensions among you, but that you be perfectly united in one mind and in one judgment."

There's another aspect to this.

Like TV's Judge Judy, my wife is a wise and practical woman, in touch with her standard of values, capable of weighing evidence and reaching sound decisions, and doing so in the heat of controversy. On the fly, if need be.

Whereas I vacillate, hem and haw between "on the one hand" and "on the other."

This is why, when the kids ask me for stuff, or to do stuff, the best answer is almost always, "Ask your mother." She'll not only know the answer, she'll be able to say it without equivocation. Even if I think I know the answer, I may be too spineless or conciliatory to say it.

Now this is not necessarily a bad thing. I know my limitations, and the kids know them, too. If it was just the three of us, we'd be living in a chaotic house, without rules. But we all three know that Mother Knows Best, she makes the rules and will enforce them.

That creates order in the home, as well as harmony, domestic tranquility.

Yes, the kids sometimes challenge the rightness of her decisions, though in the end they know she will prevail. I have learned not to challenge, not only because I know she will win, but because I know she is right.

She decides, and I abide by her decisions.

A final note: Right now there's a point of contention between my wife and me, concerning something I want to do, which will cost money, and which she opposes. She's right on principle and practicality.

And yet, I've been pleading my case, being as persuasive as I can, and recently she emailed back to me, "You're getting to me."

So she will entertain my objections, and listen. And she may even alter her decision in my favor. But, ultimately, I know, and she knows, and we all know, that it will no longer be my decision at that point, but hers.

She's the decider, I'm the abider.

Comments:

Anonymous: Now that my wife makes the final decisions, life is so much better than when there always seemed to be a power struggle. I love my wife and worship her partly because she is so much wiser than I when it comes to decisions of a relationship or social matters.

Mark: Isn't that remarkable? Me, too. It's not just that I'm a doormat and she's pushy. This thing evolved because her decisions are always superior. She has considered more factors, done so at blazing CPU speed, and especially weighed all the human factors, how a decision will affect all concerned.

and then arrived at her answer.

And apparently my wife is not unique in this. I hear it again and again. Are all women thus gifted or are we gifted in marrying especially well?

Enoch: I agree 100% on this. My wife also makes great decisions, taking every factor into account (including my wishes), and she doesn't give in. I'm thinking more and more that this is a very common trait for women.

HOH & WLM (3.10.09)

The *Sacramento Bee* recently ran an opinion piece by a part-time documentary filmmaker, William Preston Robertson,* titled "Head of Household? Let's Talk to my Wife".

(* Mr. Robertson is identified below his op-ed as "a writer, filmmaker and well-kept man who lives in Sacramento.")

The crux of the piece:

"I'm proud of my wife. She is the breadwinner in the family. She's a brilliant, dynamic, powerful woman. She works incredibly long hours and is compensated for that in a way that your average ukulele documentarian could never hope to be.

"But when my wife and I file our taxes or apply for loans, the computers, by default, make me the head of the household and my wife the 'spouse.' And they do this despite all of the usable data being located in her section of the form and all of the goose eggs being located in mine.

"I find this annoying… because it bestows upon me an un-earned status and it robs my wife of a status she has not only earned, but worked hard to attain. And as I've previously mentioned, bizarre as it may be, I'm proud of my wife.

"We live in a society that presumes in subtle and not-so-subtle ways that men are and should be the breadwinners in a household and that any other arrangement is wrong and shame-ful."

I had the same feeling of annoyance, plus awkwardness and

inauthenticity, when my wife and I went to our tax guy last month and I was given a tax return to sign as "Taxpayer" while my wife signed as "Spouse."

This after my wife, the obvious CFO (and CEO) of our family, did all the talking, responded to all the questions, produced all the documents with explanatory comments, from mortgage interest to charitable deductions, conducted a sidebar conversation with the tax guy's loan expert on doing a refi of our house. I said almost nothing, a couple of jokes, really, and was acknowledged only occasionally out of politeness by our tax guy.

Like the filmmaker, I'm proud of my wife and her leadership. What's wrong with wives being the head of their household and family? Aren't they almost always, in fact if not in name? Isn't it about time that they be allowed to take that pride of place?

Now I'll climb down from my mini-soapbox (my version of an op-ed) and, as is my wont, let some other loving female authoritarians and happily led husbands do the rest of the talking:

"We both would like to try out the 'female head of household' concept," a Norwegian husband writes to Emily Addison, the better half of the "Around Her Finger" team. "Two HOH's in a home is one too many, and I think my wife is the better manager. Serving her and taking on much more of the domestic chores are only fair, and if I can be wrapped around her finger - that is all the better."

Sounds pretty mainstream to me. As does this sensible husband: "My wife has been essentially Head of Household since we were married twenty years ago. She was a Navy officer and I an enlisted man, and to say she is smarter than I am is an understatement. Valedictorian of her high school class, and so on. Since the beginning, she has controlled the finances and many more aspects of the marriage. I'm not submissive, in fact by many measures I am a man's man. But I have come to nearly worship my wife."

"My wife is unquestionably the leader of our marriage," agrees another wife-worshipper, "but she tries her best to show me how much she appreciates my role as her husband. It's like she controls me without having to be bossy or bitchy, and I know deep in my heart that I would die for her if I had to." By the way, this guy's cyber-name is "Mr. Jenny."

Most female-led hubbies don't object to a bit of bossiness, even a superabundance thereof. On their above-mentioned blog, Emily Addison, speaking for husband Ken, recommends a candidate wife-leader assume a clear authoritarian tone: "We believe that an open and ongoing acknowledgment of the wife's authority combined with orgasm management are the fundamentals of a successful female-led relationship... You are entitled to consider his requests and then accept or dismiss them as you see fit. You are the head of household, you make the rules, and you set the guidelines... period, end of story."

Usually it is the husband who proposes the wife be HOH, less often the wife. Even less frequent are those idyllic matches when the marriage role reversal is by mutual consent from the get-go:

One guy, signed "Obedient Husband," told LFA psychologist Elise Sutton that both he and his bride agreed during their engagement that she should be undisputed head of household and take the lead "sexually, socially, emotionally, and fiscally. I regard her authority completely without question... I have been very happy in our three years together and would not seek to change a thing."

Another wife informs Ms. Sutton that her husband "recognized from the beginning that both my native intelligence and career ambitions were superior to his own and he willingly conceded to my preeminence as Head of Household. It was thus with relative ease that our marriage soon settled into its essentially Matriarchal pattern that enabled me to launch my own legal career—and also helped establish the First Rule of Our Relationship: We discuss; I decide; he obeys. In cases where my mind is already made up, or I feel strongly about a particular issue, the need for discussion is obviated and [he] is simply informed. This eliminates the need for discussion in about seventy percent of all cases, allows [him] to concentrate on his career and leaves other issues in my far more capable hands."

The marriage of "Mr. Louise" to "Mrs. Louise," described on the old Spouseclub message board, epitomizes living this lifestyle to the hilt: "We were fully aware of our roles before we walked down the aisle. I took her name. No, not secretly and not just on paper. We walked into our reception as Ms. and Mr. D. (her name) and I've never looked back. Our union is wife-centered and wife led. She is the authority I recognize and submit to and in turn she loves, cherishes and supports me. Our friends know just what I mean when I jokingly say I am under her skirt and that our marriage is 'a petticoat government.' They can see her obvious maternal/matriarchal control over our house and accept us."

Another female-empowerment psychologist, Paige Harrison, also advocates the matriarchal aspect of the wife-leader: "The Woman as the Matriarch in a love relationship can redefine family and romantic attachments. Many males tell me their strong desire to live with their Wife as the Head of Household and Domestic Disciplinarian. The Mommy-child relationship works especially well If your Wife is an extremely Maternal Woman."

And this final amen on the subject from an old standby, Au876: "More and more women are becoming the head of their households. I am proud to follow my wife's lead with my service, my actions and my heart. I may often disagree with her when we reach a fork in the road, but when she makes her decision it becomes mine and I devote myself to making it work."

Comments:
Anonymous: It would be great to read more about men taking their wife's last name. Many FLR couples aren't kinky but instead are couples where the wife is better educated and has a higher-paying job and the man may work in a lesser-paying construction job and appreciates his wife. Many construction guys i know [who are definitely not wimps] get home before their professional wives who work in an office. They younger ones don't think anything of cooking dinner and doing housework before their wives come home.

10

THE PRICE OF PEACE

Battle of Sexes Over—She Wins! (4.30.08)

"We're both more comfortable now in our proper roles."—a husband newly converted to the female-led lifestyle

That might sound like an odd comment about an extremely unconventional, role-reversal lifestyle, but it's true. Certainly for me and my wife, and I bet for many, many others. As my wife and I internalize more and more aspects of our FLR, I find that, despite the usual daily quota of conflicts, our interactions become easier. And we become more contented and "comfortable in our proper roles," just like the guy says up there. There is less friction, less rivalry, more mutual enjoyment.

Last night, for instance, in between bugging our son to do, and then keep doing his homework, I took a few minutes to leave him at the dining room table and sit down next to my wife in the living room, where she was catching up on office work while watching our daughter practice music.

She looked around to see what I wanted. I just smiled at her, a kind of goofy smile. It took her only a second to realize why I was there. Just because I wanted to be close to her, if even briefly. We had a romantic moment in that eye contact, stolen from the kids and our hectic routines.

My wife knows how I feel about her, and it's always there between us. a calm. emotional undertone. I know she feels the same way... well. not quite the same. because her love now has a special quality of accepting my devotion and worship. our special little secret.

Like that memorable exchange between Han Solo and Princess Leia from *The Empire Strikes Back*. just before he's dragged into the freezing chamber:

HAN: I love you.
LEIA: I know.

And that dialogue works for us. In fact. we've duplicated it. without meaning to quote. It comes from who we are to each other.

So. yes. far from being weird or alternative. I find that my wife and I really can be ourselves in a female-led relationship. We're much more comfortable than we were even a few years ago. when we were still trying to balance the tricky dynamics of who decides what. with occasional flareups and temper tantrums (mostly on my part).

For most couples. even long-married ones. the battle of the sexes is never quite over. It percolates at some level. maybe with half-humorous. sitcom-type gibes. trading insults and quips in front of friends. But not at our house. At our house. in our marriage. the battle of the sexes is over. and we've got a declared winner.

It's my wife. And me? I'm the lucky loser!

When the wife takes over. and the husband lets himself be lovingly led. the benefits are substantial and mutual. One wife puts it this way:

"Surprisingly. I found that my taking over the reins smoothed out some of the rough edges in our relationship and stopped some of the bickering we used to engage in. It certainly calmed [my husband] down. This led to more control in our sexual relationship. which has had even more positive results."

Comments:

Anonymous: Love your blog, but you reversed the *Empire Strikes Back* quote. Leia said "I love you" and Han said "I know." Later, in *Return of the Jedi*, the lines are reversed in another scene.

Mark: Anonymous, how could I have botched such a famous exchange? But of course you are right, and I thank you, belatedly, for setting the record straight.

Avoiding the 'S' Word — Part 1 (5.21.08)

In previous postings here and in my book, I describe the power imbalance in wife-worship marriages as a recreation of the classic rituals of courtship, where the suitor is figuratively, and often literally, on his knees before the object of his affection:

In FLRs, or female-led relationships, the power transfer is done in favor of the woman. And, since we're clearly talking about consensual relationships, that means the man has voluntarily ceded some of his power or authority over to the woman, to create an imbalance that both partners may find stimulating.

"Right now I am really feeling her power over me."

The quote is from Au876, one of the mainstays of Lady Misato's original husbands' forum on Yahoo. He goes on: "Guess I better go iron her blouse and maybe find some surprise chore to complete that she will notice."

This shows the kind of provocative imbalance that can exist between worshipped wife and worshipping husband, another aspect of the queen-knight paradigm. The queen has merely to enter the room and her knight-courtier is instantly alert to serve her in some way. ("The Power Transfer" in Chapter 9.)

Yes, I know. There are more obvious, and far-less-flattering labels that can be applied to "courtly" or "chivalrous" husbands. For example: "milquetoasts," "wimps," "wusses," "pussy-whipped" and "henpecked." I attempted to deal with these and similar putdowns in my book and in another blogpost ("Pecked & Whipped." Chapter 5).

But I seem to have tiptoed around the worst slur of all. the "S" word—for "submissive."

There's good reason for that. of course. If the husband in a wife-worship marriage is nothing more than a thinly disguised "submissive." that means the wife is just a plain old "dominant." And suddenly we are right back in the old D/s world with "Dommes" and "subs." only a sidestep away from B&D and S&M-Land. with all the whips and chains. leather and latex.

And the whole point of the recent acronymic upgrade to LFA. or Loving Female Authority. and FLR. or Female Led Relationships. was to escape that mondo bizarro ghetto. and to go mainstream with an ultra-romantic "female-led" dynamic.

And thus far. I'd say. the FLR/LFA repositioning has been amazingly successful.

So "submissive" is definitely not the noun or adjective of choice for us... well. us. uh. female-led but exceedingly macho guys.

On a message board identified with Barbara Abernathy's Venus on Top Society. renamed the "She Makes the Rules" message board. some male posters seem to exude verbal testosterone. They brag that they are captains of industry. or retired Marines. black belts. cage-fighters. and so on. Anything but submissive.

They just like to. you know. cater to assertive women... behind closed doors. of course.

Even the above-quoted Au876. a passionate advocate of the wife worship lifestyle. could go to ludicrous lengths to escape the "S" label. as in this posting:

"Someone said we were submissive husbands. I do worship and adore my wife. I will do anything she tells me (she loves me so she doesn't make me do bad things). I do all the housework. all the cooking. I take care of her. perform personal chores for her. run her errands. I put her first in everything I do. I look for ways to serve her and to show her my devotion. Her word is the law. She has complete control over all our assets and is free to do as she pleases while I am only free to do as she pleases. But you know, if someone asked me 'Are you submissive?' I would tell them no. I don't feel submissive. I feel devoted. I don't feel bossed around, I feel honored. I don't feel controlled, I feel guided and loved. Are we submissive men? Or are we men who know our place in life and are lucky enough to have a wife who cherishes us as we fulfill that place?"

Doth he not protest way too much? If that's not the life of a perfectly submissive husband he just described there, I don't know what is.

But is he wrong, and are other guys (like me) wrong, in scrupulously avoiding being branded with the flaming "S" word? (Excuse the kinky metaphor.)

Comments solicited, but more thoughts will follow in the next posting.

Comments:

Whipped One: Enjoying the dialog on the "S" word. Am I submissive? I don't know. What I do know is that when I put my wife's needs and wants above mine, I am honoring and cherishing her like I promised to do in my wedding vows.

"Husbands, take the time to talk to and more importantly listen to your wives and what they are asking you for and then act on it. I will end by saying that even if we do not have an FLR, me making my wife the #1 priority in my life absolutely cannot be negative in any way, shape or form. So instead of worrying about defining rigid roles in the relationship I am going to choose to make her a priority, give her a massage and foot rub, do housework, run errands, etc. simply because I love her and it is the right thing to do.

Mark: W.O., I especially like your point about honoring and cherishing on a daily basis as a carrying out of the promises you made in your wedding vows. That's how I first gravitated into this lifestyle, as I realized how far I had let myself slip from those promises, how much I had turned the page on courtship and was taking my wife for granted... and that I wanted and needed to get back to that.

Avoiding the 'S' Word — Part 2 (5.22.08)

In sprucing up its image. the FLR (Female Led Relationship) movement has tended to avoid terms with kinky or bizarre overtones. So. husbands or boyfriends in FLRs often resort to euphemistic synonyms for "submissive"—for example. "attentive." "accommodating." "considerate." "chivalrous." "deferential." "obliging."

Anything but submissive.

I've been one of these euphemizers. For good reason. I think. Some of my postings. as a consequence. may convey a sense of less than full disclosure.

But I begin to notice a counter movement in the world of FLRs. from guys especially. married or otherwise. who are up front about using the "S" word. Openly "submissive husbands" and "submissive boyfriends."

In fact. I'm seeing stirrings of "Submissive Pride." There's a blog called "Yes. I'm a Submissive Man!" where each posting ends with a rallying cry. "I am submissiveProud."

What's next. "Submissive Pride" marches? I don't think so. except perhaps as a subset of Gay Pride events. replete with the off-putting paraphernalia of stable and kennel. I'm afraid that's not the way back to the social mainstream. but rather deeper into the subculture swamps.

Nonetheless. some husbands in FLRs are trying to come to grips with the "S" word. like this thoughtful guy: "I myself struggle with my political beliefs in democracy and equality and my desire to serve and submit to my wife. It is hard to reconcile these two seemingly opposed impulses."

Another offers this candid insight: "Part of my thrill is the denial. the humiliation. the power trip for my wife. I like the idea of inherent unfairness. unreasonableness. inequality: for example. my wife controls all the money and can do pretty much whatever she wants. I. on the other hand. always have to ask for permission for my non-routine purchases. She can have me pleasure her to multiple orgasms, then she can roll over and fall asleep. She can masturbate anytime she wants to. I, on the other hand, need her permission before I can even touch myself for any purpose other than cleaning. The bottom line is: Her control makes me happy."

And this husband has attempted to codify his submissive status as part of an MOU (Memorandum Of Understanding) between him and his leader-wife:

"I accept the inequality inherent in a relationship based upon my erotic need to submit to my wife's will. Therefore, though I will talk to her about my thoughts and feelings, I will not try to limit her in the exercise of the prerogatives of power."

There are, to be sure, avowedly matriarchal marriages, in which the husband cannot pretend he is anything but completely submissive and subordinate, whether or not his matriarch-wife chooses to disclose their lifestyle to others.

Here's a typical example: "Before we got married, my girlfriend explained to me how she would be in total control, and she sure wasn't kidding. Now that she's my wife, she wants me to have a submissive attitude toward her at all times, not just during sex. She started asking me to do more and more housework and has become generally more and more assertive with me. We get along really well because there is no power struggle. She has begun training me to help me maintain a habit of reflexive obedience without letting my brain or ego get in the way."

"My wife reprimanded me the other day for doing something without asking permission," writes another husband. "I stated that I thought she didn't want to be bothered with that level of detail. She looked at me as if to say 'you silly man,' then she said, 'You are mine and I expect you to ask permission before you act on anything not already approved or directed.'"

I doubt that most wives in FLR marriages would want that degree of micromanagement over their husbands. But, more often than not, the degree of wifely control and of husbandly submission will be up to her to determine.

And what about the husband's part? Well, it's up to him to …

well, to oblige... and accommodate... and defer... and yield... and, okay, dammit, to submit!

I "yield" the last word to Au876:

"Abide by her decisions. Do not argue with her. Never question her but strive to make her decisions work just as you would do for your boss where you work. She is in control. Adore her and work for her."

Comments:

Burnsie: My wife has been having me shave her legs and this week (I volunteered) she is having me paint her toe- and fingernails. But she wants me to do it on the beach when we start vacation this coming weekend.

Mark: Those are very special and intimate rituals. Thus far, however, I have not been favored to shave my wife's legs—she prefers to do that in the shower. And manicures are done professionally. That leaves pedicures, however, with only occasional spa pedicures displacing my efforts.

Burnsie: I am loving the bonding that results from this. All of this is coming about very naturally, although it would still be considered "stealth" mode, as I haven't brought up FLR... yet.

john: I author the blog. Yes, I'm a submissive man! you mentioned in your post and made the decision to add "I am submissiveProud" after each post following a remarkable date with a dominant woman.

Men who are submissive—and proud of it—should be free to identify themselves as such and not worry about what others think. I'm a strong secure submissive man who thinks bowing to the authority and command of a strong dominant woman makes sense and is the right choice for me.

Mark: john, I hope you don't mind my citing your motto. It remains a goal for me to reach that state where my submissiveness can be "open, acknowledged and appreciated."

11

POWER OF THE PURSE

Direct Report to the Boss Lady (10.21.08)

In my book's last chapter, "Happy-Ever-Aftering Takes Work," I quoted wives and husbands who steer clear of arguments over money by the simple expedient of having the wife assume complete financial control.

It works, to promote not only domestic harmony but fiscal responsibility, judging from a great deal of testimony, from both genders. In that sense, according to one admittedly improvident husband, "men may well be the biggest beneficiaries" of these fiduciary arrangements.

As this wife of a spendthrift explains, "My husband has never signed his own paycheck and freely admits to anyone who will listen that he would have it no other way. Because without me in charge he would be in the poorhouse or a destitute alcoholic. Some men should never handle funds. All major spending is discussed between us, then decided on by me. He gets monies when I think he needs it."

Of course, not all wife-led marriages adhere to this strict prescription. Many chief-executive wives prefer to have their husbands remain chief financial officers, or chancellors of the exchequer. But judging from postings on FLR message boards over the years, more and more couples are opting for the power of the purse over the wallet.

Here's how it works. according to Ken Addison's popular introductory book to wife-led marriages. *Around Her Finger*: "Ideally. the household finances should be consolidated and managed by the woman. The husband should operate under a budget that she approves. and he can appeal to his wife for exceptions to that budget."

Fumika Misato goes into a little more detail on her "Real Women Don't Do Housework" website. strongly advocating this system to wives starting out in the lifestyle:

"As head of the household. you control the family finances. He is required to justify his expenses to you. But there is absolutely no need for you to explain anything whatsoever about the family finances to him. If you give him a budget it is his duty to follow it: if you require approval for certain purchases. he must obtain such approval. You. on the other hand. are free to spend as you alone see fit whether. in your judgment. for the benefit of the family or merely for your own enjoyment. For example. if you want to buy a new car. that is your decision alone. but if he wants to purchase a new shirt he must seek your permission."

One of Lady Misato's faithful followers. Au876. described how this dynamic operated in his wife-led marriage: "My wife now has total control of all our assets. My check goes by direct deposit into her account. and I am given an allowance which she sets and adjusts as she sees fit. I am not allowed nor do I ever question any decisions she makes about finances (or anything else for that matter)."

How. one may ask. does this unequal status reflect the courtship ideal inherent in wife-worship? It may be a stretch. but I really think it's there. Work with me here. as they say on sitcoms. and conjure up the knight errant returning to court and laying some trophy of battle (the Holy Grail. perhaps?) at the feet of his queen or lady fair.

Or picture a caveman returning to his cave and throwing down his bloody kill at the feet of his cavelady. Perhaps he had to carve off a cutlet or two to eat en route. but I assure you he'd have preferred to lay the carcass intact at her feet. That's the thrill of manly service to the she-creature who rules his heart.

That's the same hard-wired macho impulse, slightly twisted, that has guys emptying their wallet onto the railings of strip club stages on Friday nights.

But, as I said, there are other working and workable FLR arrangements, some of which give the husband more discretion in family finances.

"In our house," one husband explains, "it's my job to keep up with the finances. My wife is the breadwinner and of course she has the final decision how the money is to spent. The way it works is I keep the books and if she wants to know some details, I report to her. I have some money for my personal needs, so I don't have to ask her or keep track of those expenditures."

Another husband can buy whatever he likes without wifely permission, until he reaches a hundred-dollar threshold: "My Wife and I are both accountants, so it wasn't a problem when about a month ago she decided to assume full financial control as part of her role of having final authority in our marriage. She decided I will receive a weekly allowance of cash from her to use any way I wish, but I need to get Her advance permission on any purchases over $100. I'm not allowed to write any checks or making any savings withdrawals from our bank accounts."

An interesting variation on these arrangements is where the wife controls the finances but relies on her husband for financial advice, keeping the books and handling all relevant paperwork. She just makes the decisions and signs the checks.

As Ken Addison puts it in *Around Her Finger*: "If, as a practical matter, the wife feels that she wants to defer the administrative component of managing the money (*e.g.* balancing a checkbook), then she can delegate this task as she would any other. If she decides to delegate this task, however, it is important that she get regular and frequent updates on the status of income and expenses in the home."

Fdhousehusband (of the discontinued blog "her househusband's life") again gives some personal details: "In Her

Household, my Wife earns almost all the money but i pay all the bills. i am really more of just Her secretary though. i prepare a budget every year that She then reviews and approves... i am to stay within the budget and advise Her whether proposed spending is within the budget. She can always change the budget and like a good secretary my job is to just advise Her of the choices She has to make."

Another husband describes a variation of the same matriarchal management theme: "The money is my wife's, but one of my duties is to be the accountant. She is President and CEO, and as an underling, I make regular financial reports to let her know how her finances stand. As for big ticket items (cars, vacations, etc.) She has me do extensive research on all the possibilities. She will have me give a presentation to her, briefly going through pros, cons, options, etc. In the end, though, she makes the final choice, regardless of whether I thought it was the very best one or not."

Au876 is also privileged to be his wife's financial advisor, financial secretary and, ultimately, accounts payable clerk: "Bill-paying is a chore as are many other aspects of financial management. I get all the bills ready for payment and she signs the checks. My wife often has me gather information on an investment she may be considering or do other research, such as comparing prices, etc. She often asks my opinion. When she does, she expects an informed opinion. However, after I present what she has asked for, she makes the decisions. Sometimes I never know what they are, but I have been asked for an opinion and that by itself thrills me."

It was a decade ago in Lady Misato's Wife Worship Forum that I first read Au876's description of his wife's stringent financial control. So I asked him, deeply puzzled, how he could buy his wife any special or expensive presents for Valentine's or Christmas or birthdays without funds. His answer came as a revelation:

"This is in reply to your question of how I could buy my wife expensive gifts. I can't. There is no way possible because I do not have free access to any remotely large sum of money. If she wants something, she buys it and I must say she does not hesitate to splurge on herself. Before she took control of the finances I would buy her expensive gifts from time to time. She appreciated them but often exchanged them for what she really wanted. Now she buys what she really wants. But the big plus is how much more she appreciates the gifts I do buy for her. It may be an inexpensive sweater, some new underwear, candy or even flowers from time to time, but she knows I have had to save back from my allowance to make the purchase and she knows I have given up some pleasures for myself to please her. She seems to appreciate them much more than she did expensive gifts that caused me little hardship."

I was deeply impressed by the extent of Au876's devotion. Now, after many years, I am privileged to confirm from my own daily experience the truth of what he wrote:

"There are very few things you can do without money. If your wife controls the money, she largely controls what you can and cannot do. Meanwhile, she can do what she wants with no approval or permission from you."

Yes, it's a primal thrill for any wife-worshipper to relinquish all financial power into the hands of his queen, but I will whisper one teensy-weensy caution that others in the life have passed on to me:

Be careful what you wish for. Giving up financial control may be a point of no return on the road to wifedom.

Where Have You Gone, Nancy and Dennis? (8.13.08)

A couple of years back, on the old Yahoo "Venus on Top Discussion Board" (now evolved into the "She Makes the Rules Discussion Board"), there appeared a series of provocative and strongly worded posts on the dynamics and advantages of wife-led marriages.

The messages were signed "Nancy and Dennis" (though apparently all written by Dennis). a couple who. by their own description. not only advocated but evangelized for female-led relationships.

Alas. after several weeks. the Nancy-and-Dennis dispatches stopped and appeared no more. Since then. I've found no evidence of them elsewhere in cyberspace.

Where have you gone. Nancy and Dennis? And are Ms. and Mr. Lynda of the old Spouseclub with you? Please come back or drop us a line. I'm sure there are many enthusiasts for this wonderful lifestyle who would welcome an update on your happy wife-led marriage.

In the meantime. here is a short sampling from their old old posts. grouped into a few topics (with apologies to the moderators of the former VOT Board):

Their Backstory

"Nancy and I have been in a female-led situation for over 25 years. Nancy is in charge of our household. She manages our finances. makes all major decisions. and sets our social agenda. Nancy's mother. Sue. lives with us and I defer to her as I would Nancy...

"[But] while both Nancy and her mother can be quick-tempered. ours is not a BDSM relationship. nor am I going about the house teetering on heels with a feather duster when doing housework. Ours is a pragmatic relationship with a variety of house rules and expectations where my opinions are valued and considered. In the end. of course. we all recognize that women will be making the final decisions!"

"Nancy and I met in college—at a NOW meeting no less—and hit it off quickly. Nancy assumed a leadership role right from the start and that role continues to this day. Over the years she's taken more power. She's the financial manager and decision maker who is focused on her career. I. on the other hand.

do the majority of the housework and am generally supportive of Nancy's career and personal goals. Socially, we enjoy the company of other couples who, like us, are in varying degrees of female-led relationships."

"We work at a local women's center where we conduct workshops aimed at getting women to be more assertive in their personal relationships... We offer them practical tips for taking control, the first of which is for women to take control of the finances."

"We are evangelists for female-dominated relationships and want to encourage more couples to embark on them. We advise women to take control of their relationships and do so by becoming more demanding of their men. These three points—money, housework, and social life—emerge as the big ones."

"What women want, in our experience, is some say in the finances, a man who'll bear his share of the housework, and a man that she can share social activities with. In our view women can't have too much control of these important relationship elements."

FLR = Harmony & Happiness
"Nancy and I do have differences of opinion but my opinion is sought and considered, although we all recognize that within our relationship women will be making the final decision and, once made, that decision is final."

"Our opinion is that female-led relationships have fewer issues and problems than vanilla ones, but this assumes that an FLR is a total commitment, not just a game. It also assumes benevolence on the part of the woman making the decisions in that relationship."

"As a man I can tell you that I like knowing exactly what my wife wants and when and how she wants it done. No conflict; no arguments. And I can tell you that most men really do want to make their wives happy."

POWER OF THE PURSE

Financial Control

"Nancy and I teach that managing finances is critical to a woman's leading a relationship. [Women] might want to enhance [their] skills in this area by seeking a skilled financial planner and or taking some workshops. Women's organizations such as NOW and the YWCA are good places to start for such resources."

"I'm embarrassed to say that I was quite the spendthrift early in our marriage and spending money and not able to account for it, so Nancy put her foot down and initiated some pretty strict rules. She took away my debit card, limited how much money I could have with me at any one time – I was spending WAY too much at work buying coffee, lunches, and so on for too many people, too often.

"Her rules include limiting me to an allowance (albeit a generous one), requiring direct depositing of my paychecks, her having access to my company savings and benefits plans, limiting my use of bank and credit cards, and requiring justification of all card charges.

"How I spend my allowance is up to me but I've made a habit of asking Nancy's opinion on larger purchases. I can request [extra funds] but there are almost always conditions attached. Having to ask for money is a tremendous statement of who is in control. We are now financially solid as a result of her controls."

House Rules

"We have a number of practical house rules that we've established over the years, mostly things that have just evolved from practice as opposed to being dictates from my wife. Discipline is rare; I understand her expectations and, for the most part, meet them...We are friends with other couples in similar situations – households where the men realize the innate superiority of the women and defer to them."

199

Power Exchange

"[Women shouldn't] feel guilty about using power. Men derive tremendous benefits from an FLR so women should use the power they derive from such a relationship and seek more of it...

"In our evangelization of this lifestyle we frequently cite our own and the experiences of couples we know in FLR situations. All are extremely happy and wouldn't want it any other way. But it takes specifics to get things rolling one small step at a time. Once the lifestyle has momentum though, our experience is that he'll be doing more, offering more power on his own."

That's all, alas, for now. But why not check out the workshop offerings at your local women's center? You just might find Nancy and Dennis bringing their evangelizing act to a venue near you.

Comments:
Norman: There doesn't seem to be much by way of public figures openly endorsing FLM. Granted, there are women in the field (many of whom you refer to or quote regularly), but it would be nice to see more people openly evangelizing female led-relationships.

Mark: Well said. One of the attractions of the Nancy-Dennis posts was that they were written by a husband who presented himself as a spokesperson for FLRs, or FLMs, a man who, in tandem with his wife, regularly made public presentations on the benefits of female-led relationships at YWCAs and other community venues.

Not a prominent or public figure, but at least a man going public. And I thought, as I read these posts, that this just might be the leading edge of a movement—along with Barbara Abernathy's public appearances on behalf of her website and book. Not a good sign that Dennis and his Nancy seem to have gone back underground.

Norman: There's kind of a catch-22 going on. Women who would openly endorse it end up looking like (or I should say being branded as) control-freak bitches. And guys would either run the risk of major ridicule, or grabbing the spotlight in a way that sounds oxymoronic—*i.e.*, he should be in a supporting role for her, not the star.

12

DEGREES (AND DECREES) OF DOMESTICITY

Bedtime Stories (11.26.08)

Let me tell you about a good friend of mine who married a gorgeous blonde. A Candy Bergen/Catherine Deneuve-class blonde. I kid you not. He was a compulsive late-night person, while she went to bed early. I told him, right after the honeymoon, that he should change his ways pronto. I mean, a no-brainer, right?

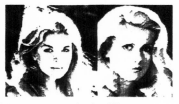

But he never did, and the marriage unraveled. There were plenty of other persuasive reasons cited, but I always wondered what would have happened if my friend had just made it a policy to put down his post-adolescent toys whenever his bride was ready for bed and gone to play with her instead.

Many years later I finally got hitched... and forgot my advice. Not always, but too frequently I would stay up after she retired, playing with the computer or watching sports.

Then I discovered wife worship—just in time, thank God! And there I discovered my old bedtime dictum emblazoned as one of the cardinal rules. In fact, I have yet to come across an example cited by any female-led couple where it is otherwise.

Here is a typical example of the benefits of synchronized bed-times, from a recent Internet friend who shares the wife-worship lifestyle:

"One of the things I did before with my obsessive hobby was stay up way too late after [my wife] went to bed. Since our rec-onciliation, I make a point of going to bed at the same time as her. When we go upstairs, while she is in the bathroom, I will turn over the bedcovers and fluff up her pillow. This past week, I have made a point of leaving a small Peppermint Patty on the pillow. When she comes in the room, if she is not already changed for bed, I help her change. I help pull off her jeans and panties, unhook her bra, and fold her clothes neatly over the chair. I help her into her nightie. When we get into bed, I usually offer her a backrub."

And we fade out...

Bedtime for Bonzo

Why doesn't every husband follow this recipe for nocturnal togetherness? Granted, it isn't easy to change longtime bio-rhythmic patterns. Often, it seems, it takes a resolute wife to takes matters into her own hands and imposes a curfew on a time-philandering husband.

fdhousehusband (who, alas, is on extended vacation from his own FLR blog, "Her househusband's life") is fortunate enough to belong to just such a wife:

"i was always a night person before i became Her househus-band, but after a while i began to be in sync with my morning person Wife. She requires that i go to bed before 11:00 pm ('my curfew,' She calls it) and that helps me wake up without an alarm clock. i don't drink coffee as She forbids me from having caffeine. ('You don't need caffeine to motivate you, that is My job,' She says)."

Here's another guy taken in hand by his wife: "My wife be-gan dictating that i would no longer stay up watching tv but would go to bed when she went to bed and wake at a specified time, early to get ready for work, deal with the children, and get breakfast started."

And another:

"Every night, I was required to go to bed at the same time as my wife, and stroke her body while she went to sleep. On about half of all nights she would become sexually excited while I stroked her skin and proceed to have orgasms, assisted by vibrators, or my oral or manual ministrations..."

My night-owl friend would certainly have profited from a take-charge wife like those, or this one: "I gave my husband a curfew for coming to bed nightly so that he wasn't up all night watching sports or God knows what. Bedtime is either 10 or 10:30. He has different duties each night. Some nights it's a massage, some nights he pleases me with oral sex. Some nights we just cuddle."

Cuddle Time

Cuddling and footrubs are pretty much standard features of these romantic bedtime stories. I offer typical excerpts:

"My favorite part of the day is bedtime," a husband explains, "when i massage her feet with lotion and kiss them and we talk about our day and, if I'm lucky, cuddle. This has become a nightly ritual that we both enjoy."

"My wife and I go to bed together every night (unless she is out real late, in which case I am already in the bed). I make a point of this. I am never first (well hardly never) to go to bed. When she goes, I go. Then, after I rub her feet with lotion, almost always I cuddle with her and tell her how much I love and adore her. I do this for as long as she will allow."

"My husband's nightly routine begins by placing a glass of water beside the bed, turning down the sheets and waiting for me to arrive. Once I am in bed, he gives me a 10-15 minute foot rub to help me relax and get ready to sleep. I feel completely pampered and taken cared of, and my husband feels wonderful that he can serve me and worship me in this manner."

"I am expected to prepare the Queen's bedroom for Her at bedtime, lighting candles, warming Her pajamas for Her, and choosing music to fit Her mood. I must request entry into Her bed, where I perform nightly massage and can be awakened at any time when She needs attention."

"In a little while, i will rub Her feet before bedtime. (She alone will decide if I go right to sleep or if She wants sex tonight). i am very happy in our lifestyle."

"When she's ready to go to bed, I go up with her and rub her back, legs and feet until she's asleep. She now expects me to do this, which makes me VERY happy, and says she can't go to sleep without it! When she falls asleep I go downstairs to do a few minor chores (fold more laundry, clean up the living areas, recharge her cell phone, whatever)."

"We both know that I'll be pampering her when we go to bed. Makes for a pretty nice life—for both of us."

"When we go to bed at night i kiss Her feet and service Her orally if She wants. my sexual activity is totally under Her control and i am not allowed to touch myself without Her permission."

"my Wife told me to come to bed. i rested the side of my head in Her left underarm and curled up beside Her. She hugged me with Her right arm and placed Her right leg over my hips. i placed my right hand on Her chest..."

Some take-charge wives assume an uncompromising tone in the matter of imposing curfews for hubby:

"From being a game," one husband confides on a wife-led message board, "it's now become the default that I get ready for bed when she chooses to, kneel by her bed to await instructions (sometimes she just wants to go straight to sleep but often she wants me to pleasure her.)"

This wife even utilizes the 24-hour military clock for scheduling her mate's rising and setting: "Husband's chores must be completed before curfew. He is required to be up no later that 0900 on the days he works the later shift and his days off."

"My wife has drastically curtailed my television time," a man writes, praising her firmness, "and assigns an early bedtime if my chores are done. It is her philosophy that any distractions in a man's life must be removed in order for him to remain focused on his wife."

DEGREES (AND DECREES) OF DOMESTICITY

"Gotta hurry," another husband typed in a hasty bulletin board message. "I have only 3 minutes till bedtime."

Isn't it demeaning for a husband to be ordered to bed by his wife? Of course it is. And yet I can't help thinking that many a failed marriage (like my friend's) could have been saved by exactly such a no-nonsense maternally imposed regimen. More examples: "'Time for bedtime, sweetie,' my Wife said. 'You have a busy day tomorrow.'"

"'Go to bed now,' ordered my wife as I was completing my chores. 'You must get up at 5 a.m. tomorrow morning to serve me breakfast in bed.' A few minutes later, she joined me in bed."

"After a bit more relaxing at her feet in front of the TV, my wife made me go to bed early, telling me that tomorrow would probably be a 'big day for my little boy.' This time, her words made me feel very little and very embarrassed."

"My wife took to the female-led relationship big-time, making all the decisions, even telling me when I had to go to bed. Secretly I liked it, and I knew she could tell. I hardly put up any resistance."

Some wives, in fact, use bedtime to review hubby's daily performance, rather than wait for the Weekend Update, which is the subject of a two-part posting (see Chapter 14):

"I keep a private journal. It is closer to a daily love letter to my wife. It is my one uncensored outlet for telling her how I am feeling and what I am thinking. She usually has me read it to her as part of our bedtime ritual. I get in trouble if I have no entry for that day."

"I spent the next twenty minutes rubbing her feet. It excited the hell out of me. She could tell too. When I finished she said, 'Well, I guess you have finished most of your chores for the day. Did you clean my tennis shoes?' 'Yes.' 'Then you can go to bed now.'"

For yet other worshipped wives, sending hubby to bed early constitutes punishment for substandard performance:

"My husband neglected his chores the last two days. I have changed his bedtime to 8:15 pm until Monday."

A husband who signs himself "Mr. Mary" writes: "For me,

being made to go to bed early and not getting to watch a favorite program on TV is a punishment that can really put me in my place."

Another husband amens: "The mildest form of punishment my wife would employ is something like being sent to bed early, which i don't enjoy because i always prefer to stay up past midnight. If i argue about it, then i am forced to go to bed early and switch the light out, so that i can't read in bed."

Finally, just to sketch out the wide spectrum of bedtime behaviors in female-led relationships, here are a couple of matriarchal households in which hubby may find himself dismissed to bed in front of guests—demonstrating the wife's complete authority over him:

The first one was posted under the name of "Charles" on the now-defunct Spousechat message board: "After dinner, I made coffee for [Lisa and her friends], they went into the living room and talked business for a while, while I cleaned up. After cleaning up, I went in and politely asked 'Will there be anything else, ladies?' Lisa's guests thanked me and replied no. Lisa said 'No, that'll be all, but before you go to bed Charles, go through my closet and see if you can find that orange print skirt, you know the flowered one that I bought in St Croix last year? It'll probably need to be ironed but you can do that in the morning, just see if you can find it tonight, I want to wear it tomorrow.' 'Yes' I replied and left the room..."

"Rebecca," an unapologetic advocate of all-out matriarchy, offered wives this advice on her Yahoo! Group ("Happy Wives, Trained Husbands," also long defunct):

"Bedtime is an excellent time for husband training. Controlling what time he goes to bed, where and how he sleeps, what he wears, is excellent training because he thinks about his situation all night in his subconscious. If it is done in front of a witness he cannot deny it and cannot pretend it did not happen. For example, you have another couple over for the evening. Say to your husband, 'Dear, it's bedtime for you, go get ready and get in bed and I'll be in to check you in a few moments.' He must obey and you have shown your authority."

Better by far, guys, to just take the hint and go hand in hand with your beloved to dreamland.

Comments:
Anon: "[My wife] has given me a bedtime because I was always staying up too late and therefore too tired all the time. Now she has me in bed by 9 pm! I can read a book till 10 pm. She joins me around that time. Lately, I am reading the book *She Comes First* by Ian Kerner. She's taking very well to the concept of her managing my orgasms.

I think my wife is a gift from God. This gift however, becomes more beautiful and more valuable the more I love, honor, obey, serve, and appreciate her. I submit to my wife and I am beyond happy."

Losing His Grip (11.4.08)

In my book, *Worshipping Your Wife*, I talk about husbands losing their grip—on the TV remote control:

"...husbands ought to haul themselves off their couches en masse, relinquish their remotes and take up their honey-do lists." (Chapter 5)

"...my advice to husbands is: Find the 'Power Off' button on the remote, get off the couch and start courting your wife. (Chapter 6)

"Not a few husbands mention handing over the remote to their wives as a big-deal behavioral modification. And it *is* a big deal. Watching TV with my wife, I often find myself with a death-grip on the button-studded contraption. Like NRA card-carriers, most of us guys will give up our remotes only if they're pried out of our 'cold dead hands.' (Chapter 7)

But why, guys, is handing over the remote to our wives so difficult? Even for a moment? For some of us, endorsing the entire paycheck to her or giving up our nights out with the boys can be easier.

I'm not going to get psychoanalytical about it. You can

speculate, if you like. Let's just stipulate, as the lawyers say, that it *is* difficult. In some way, the ultimate power transfer.

Which reminds me of another quote from my book, in chapter 6, about "Meyer's Law" as codified by mystery novelist John D. MacDonald: "In all emotional conflicts, the thing you find hardest to do is the thing you should do."

Husbands who successfully unwrap their fingers from this battery-operated IR-gun report a sense of liberation, like kicking an addiction. They find, again to quote myself, "it's lots more fun to play with her in bed than with the TV remote."

Some eloquent examples:

"After we reconciled, I realized that I would much rather be with her than watch the shows I like... Because of this, she ended up as the undisputed queen of the remote control. When we came downstairs to look at television, I would pick up the remote and hand it to her, and then submit to whatever she wanted to watch. She commented the other day that I am so domesticated now that I'm watching HGTV with her, and that she never would have believed that a couple of years ago."

"Over the years, i have developed a number of routines that i now follow out of habit... [including] handing Her the TV remote. Each time i perform these little domestic routines i reinforce my supportive role in Her Life."

"When we adopted an FLR marriage," another husband explains, "the TV remote became Hers. However, the music to be played in the car had been determined by who was driving. That changed too. The car stereo is now an extension of the TV remote and She will now choose the music, regardless of who is driving or which car we are in."

"I truly love my wife and do the utmost to please her. I wasn't always like that, but now I get up before her, prepare breakfast, make up the bed and clean up while she gets ready for work. I cook and clean up. And she controls the remote on the TV."

"I rub my wife's feet every evening and give her massages whenever she wants them. And she now exclusively has the remote for the TV."

DEGREES (AND DECREES) OF DOMESTICITY

"I have handed over the TV remote. although sometimes I ask if she minds if we watch a certain show."

Many husbands realize what a big deal this "little" gesture can be:

"I realize that I am able to be defer to my wife in many subtle ways. from small things like turning over the TV remote to sitting at her feet as she reads or watches TV and massaging her feet."

"You should vigorously pursue every opportunity to give your wife massages. talk to her about things that interest her. leave the remote in her hands. fetch her something to drink. make dinner. clean up afterwards. etc."

And what about the wives? Almost without exception. those embarking on female-led relationships seem eager to wrap their lovely fingers around this particular symbol of power. recognizing it as akin to the scepter of state held by the queen:

"You will come to enjoy the freedom in decision-making afforded you." writes Emily Addison of "Around Her Finger." "If you want to be the only half of the couple allowed to use the remote control. you need only say so."

One wife. reveling in newfound domestic supremacy. ranked "I get first rights to the remote control" as No. 11 among her new perks.

I don't mean to give the impression that wife-worshipping husbands eagerly surrender the remote control. Many guys. indeed. have to have this favorite toy pried from their grips. and not always at an opportune time.

One wife chose to assert her electronic-gadget authority in the middle of "Monday Night Football." The shocked husband recounts the traumatic incident: "She turned it off. took the remote. I was stunned. 'From now on.' she said. brandishing the remote. "this is mine. You are not to touch it.'"

"We decided that from a certain date on." writes another wife on the "Around Her Finger" blog. "I would decide what TV shows he and I watched. Most of the time he was very agreeable to me changing the channel to watch what I wanted. but there were times. especially on Sunday afternoons. when I would switch to a romantic movie and force him to miss a football game. He grumbled, quietly, but he grumbled nonetheless."

In some advanced arrangements, husbands are expected to defer happily to their governing mates in all things, most definitely including channel selection: "My husband and I are believers in matriarchy," a wife explains to Elise Sutton. "At dinner, I'm the one who sits at the head of the table. While we're watching TV, I'll have him bring me a cup of coffee or a tray of fruit. Best of all, I'm in total control of the remote."

But even the most compliant guy can harbor a few frustrations as he observes occasional female ineptitude with the finer points of electronic button-pushing: "We have a complex TV setup and despite three months of gentle coaching, she keeps screwing it up. There is an element in me that feels very insecure that I've seeded control of my life to Someone who can't use a remote control."

Another husband concurs: "It still drives me crazy that she now has the universal remote control and struggles to use it... Man, I've got a long way to go."

What's a well-meaning guy supposed to do? Well, according to fdhousehusband, he should just settle back and realize that "she has the authority to make mistakes."

One couple arrived at an electronic compromise, as this husband details: "I sit at my wife's feet while she sits in the comfortable easychair. I am in charge of the remote control, but she is in charge of me."

Pavlovian Postscript: As I was getting ready to post this, I came across a quote from a husband whose wife kept two electronic remotes, one to control the TV and a second to control him:

"The power of a remote control can be used for so much more interesting endeavors than just changing channels on the television. My wife had a remote control and she would give me different sensations of pleasure and pain from the very mild electrical charges."

DEGREES (AND DECREES) OF DOMESTICITY

Comments:

Anonymous: The sight of a woman controlling a remote control and or watching TV while the husband does housework in the background or serves her drinks and food is one of the sexiest images that I can think of.

Bob: I think that if a couple want to make their FLR public, while not seeming too kinky, one good way would be for the wife to invite her friends over to watch a female-oriented show (like "Gray's Anatomy"). The husband would fix sandwiches for the ladies and serve them drinks and wash dishes in the kitchen. He would not have to overdo it, just be quiet and obedient and keep the focus on his wife's needs and her girlfriend's needs. Most women like to talk with their girlfriends without their husbands interrupting.

Mark: Bob, your comment about the wife inviting her girlfriends over to watch a woman's show and the husband helping to greet and serve and then generally stay out of the way reminded me of a favorite quote from a "Mr. Louse" on the old Spouseclub message board (archived on my blog): "The sound of male silence while women are conversing is the music of the matriarchal home."

Anonymous: One remote control a husband should be happy to let his wife use is described on the Dream Lover Labs site.

Boys Night Out, Part 1 (7.18.08)

My wife never tried to break up that old gang of mine, or put a stop to an occasional boys' nights out. I was just never one of those beer commercial guys. You know, those arrested-development homies, still wearing their caps backward and high-fiving over "Monday Night Football."

Well, maybe it was kinda like that, once upon a time. There were a few guys—quasi-nerds, mostly, but we did sorta fun stuff. Before the bonds of matrimony got tied and double-knotted. For all of us. After that, it was Life with the Wife. And Kids.

But for some husbands, apparently, bachelor shenanigans never end. The revolving poker night. Friday night at the sports bar.

For others, it's a last-minute invite as they're leaving work.

211

Hey, a bunch of the guys are heading to Hooters to watch the Big Game (and the Jiggle Parade).

Not in a wife-led marriage, though. Not with the wife in firm control—of purse strings, hubbie's schedule and to-do list. A night out with the boys, if permitted at all, will be ground-ruled and time-limited—and probably about as tame as my bachelor party (which my bride-to-be actually planned for me).

A female-led husband won't be hanging twenties on the strip-club rail, or buying a round of drinks for the table. He won't have the cash. And he'd better not use plastic, because it's her account, and she'll be scanning the statement at the end of the month, line by line. "Hooters? $58.50?"

In fact, some women take firm control even before the wedding. Like this one:

"My fiance's house was full of stupid things. I told him I planned to have a better use of our money. Of course, he will have a daily allowance, and even a credit card for emergencies, but he will need to justify all expenses. I will control his schedule. He has already curfews and I spanked him today for not coming home right after playing golf and not calling me."

"You will be in charge of the finances," another woman advises a bride about-to-be. "You will make sure you do not end up with $300 dartboards and have your husband spend $100 on a night out with the boys."

Here are a couple more wives explaining how NOWTBs (Nights Out With the Boys) have become a thing of the past:

Wife No. 1: "Theoretically, my husband could go out for a drink with a friend after work, but he does not have the ability to pay his tab so he makes excuses and comes home. He is required home by a specific time every night anyway, but if he does want to go out with a friend he simply has to clear it with me first and provide me with adequate notice so that his chores can be rescheduled. Obviously he cannot make arrangements, on the spur of the moment, as he will not have the means to pay."

Wife No. 2, you'll see, actually authorizes occasional but carefully controlled NOWTBs: "My husband commutes on the train (second class) on a season ticket whereas his colleagues go first class or drive their flashy cars and go out partying after work. He's considered henpecked but very occasionally I'll authorize him to go with them for an hour or so and buy a round of drinks, just to maintain his status. Afterward I check his wallet and, of course, check his credit card statement at month end."

"My wife decides where I spend my time and who I associate with when away from her," one tightly leashed husband confesses. "I know if I'm as much as five minutes late home from work I'd better have a good explanation. When I'm not near a phone I carry a cell phone with the power on. She can and has called to test me."

Another husband was issued a pager by his wife. Whenever she paged him, he had exactly three minutes to call in—or else!

Pager or cell phone? Either will do, according to female supremacist Julie Wilson (some of whose online writings can be found on her MySpace blog). Ms. Wilson advises husbands to "keep a pager or cell phone [in the car] so you can be called at a moment's notice."

Yet another husband was actually given a pager for home use. "Every time she needs something, she'll page me to get it for her if I'm not in the room."

That leading light of the FLR movement, Lady Misato (of "Real Women Don't Do Housework"), suggests that wives consider allowing their mates a night out with the boys as a reward for sufficiently meritorious service (estimable gifts given, chores diligently done, intimate services performed, etc.).

But husbands denied NOWTBs also benefit healthwise, as this husband realizes: "My midweek couple of beers after work drinking is really a thing of the past, and I told her that I really liked what her having control was doing for my fitness."

In FLR marriages, however, "girls nights out" seem to be frequent events, whether regularly scheduled or spur of the moment. And left-behind husbands are not to question these outings. Not where or when, not how long or with whom. "What?" is permitted only if it pertains to what chores she expects to have completed during her absence.

I kid you not. Au876 tells a tale on himself:

"[My wife] goes out a fair amount of nights. I was all excited about her coming home from work this evening. I had her favorite dinner simmering on the stove when she got home. After dinner she went to check her email while I cleaned up the kitchen. When she came down she put on her coat and started out the door, saying she was going out with a couple of her friends to a movie. She saw the disappointed look on my face. As she left, she told me not to wait up for her. Guess I better go iron her blouse and maybe find some surprise chore to complete that she will notice. One thing is for sure, I can't complain to her because that isn't allowed."

Another husband amens: "My wife and her friends often have ladies night out where the husbands stay at home with the kids or clean the bathroom."

One female supremacist goes a step farther, requiring her stay-at-home guy to help her prepare for her girls nights out. "I prefer to have him naked when he's helping me get ready... It gives it just the right feeling."

That's one aspect of boys-night-out role reversal as practiced in female-led households. There's another, equally intriguing.

Which I'll leave for the next post.

Comments:
Whatevershesays: My wife isn't that social and doesn't want to go out after work. Prefers to play with our kids. I don't seem to have the time with all the activities of keeping our house/kids running smoothly. However, I do kinda ask her when I do want to go out. It's so infrequent, she rarely says no. Our home cordless phone has a pager built in. She uses that and I come running.

Anonymous: A perfect FLR scenario would be for the women to have a girls night out while the men stayed at a different wife's house a week and cleaned it top to bottom.

DEGREES (AND DECREES) OF DOMESTICITY

Boys Night Out, Part 2 (7.22.08)

As discussed in the previous post, many in-charge wives put the clamps on their hubby's nights out with the boys, for a variety of reasons. But having done that, establishing their authority over their mate's time, some wives encourage their husbands to seek male company—of a less macho sort.

These new male companions are hand-picked by the wives, just as my bride-to-be selected the male invitees to my bachelor party. The number one criterion for the new candidates is that they also be in female-led relationships.

The idea is that any male bonding that takes place will be within the inescapable context of their mutual interest—being controlled by their respective wives.

One way of ensuring that the two husbands reinforce each other's commitment to the lifestyle, rather than indulge in a gripe session, is to have the wives present to set the agenda. And sometimes this is done, as you'll read below.

At other times, however, the husbands are allowed to interact without wifely oversight. Does this lead to mutinous masculine grumblings, hatchings plots to undermine their wives' authority?

Hardly. Almost always (judging by the online discussions I've seen) the husbands in FLRs form an ad hoc support group, comparing notes and trading tips on ways to be even more devoted and useful to their wives. Even complaining may take the form of submissive one-upmanship, each trying to top the other with stories about how strict his wife is. A typical exchange:

Househubby No. 1: "I'm going out of my tree. My wife has teased me every night and denied me orgasm for two weeks now."

Househubby No. 2: "Is that all? Try two months, like my princess does to me."

And I came across this quote from a guy boasting about his wife's "developing dominance," saying it was "intriguing and also a bit scary":

215

"For example, only this morning she said to me, 'I think I need two husbands, don't you think that would be a good idea? You're so good around the house and with the kids, but we need someone handy. Plus you could compare notes on me. Wouldn't that be fun?' Of course, she was only joking (I think)."

Online support groups fill obvious needs for both wives and husbands in FLRs—providing reinforcement, reassurance, feedback, occasional cautionary words-to-the-wise and a wealth of been-there-tried-that ideas for taking the lifestyle up a notch.

Some of these valuable FLR-related forums have vanished (Spousechat), some have migrated (Lady Misato's from Yahoo to Facebook, the Venus On Top Discussion Group to the new SheMakesTheRules message board, etc.).

Elise Sutton's Q&A resource remains in place, though in recent months she has been using recycled material on her free site (while saving fresh material for her subscription site).

All of these I have found to be, by and large, congenial gathering places, non-judgmental, with new members welcomed warmly by existing members, as in this exchange I saved from Lady Misato's original Wife Worship Forum:

Old Member: "Welcome! Get a cup of coffee, sit back and read all the posts to this forum from the beginning. You'll soon see you're not alone! Keep serving your wife, putting her first. Listen intently when she speaks and do everything she says. Encourage her to join the wives' forum as soon as she feels like it…"

New Member (replying a day later): "Thanks for the warm welcome. Having read through all of the posts on this forum (as you suggested), I have come to one conclusion that every man here feels almost exactly as i do…."

Here's how my favorite wife-worshipper, Au876, explained how much the online community of like-minded husbands meant to him:

"I too very much enjoy all the postings and knowing other husbands find joy in serving their wives. I am glad to be here and am thankful for our Founder [Lady Misato] having the grace

216

to set up a site where men on the cutting edge can discuss, exchange and even daydream. It is great to have a place where I, and we, can get it off our chest and know we are understood by those that read our post.

"For instance, I have never told anyone that my wife sometimes punishes me by making me stand in a corner or write some mundane essay for her. Yet you guys understand why I comply and don't laugh at me or consider me a wimp (I hope) for doing so."

Of course, Au876 was talking about a virtual gathering place, an online "Cheers!" bar where everybody only knows your pseudonym. A similar confession—about being stood in the corner by one's wife, say, and submitting to it—would be much more difficult, embarrassing and unlikely in an actual support group, with guys sitting around in the same room. Or even two guys, face to face.

If or until the idea of female-led marriages becomes safely mainstream, most husbands and wives will wish to keep their domestic arrangements behind closed doors.

Yet some husbands express a longing, not to be publicly "outed," but to share their experiences with other like-minded husbands—in the flesh, not just in cyberspace:

"It would be nice if I were able to develop real-life friendships with some other guys who are part of an FLR couple."

This particular househusband, however, did not think he would ever have that opportunity, because his wife was very protective of their privacy, and he dared not do this without her permission.

Some FLR couples, however, are quite up front about their role-reversal lifestyle. At restaurants, for instance, the leading wife may take the power position, dealing exclusively with the waiter, ordering for her husband, paying the check, etc. "Ms. and Mr. Lynda BJ" were one such, who posted frequently on the old Spousechat message board. Here is a description by Ms. Lynda of one such "outing," and how it led to Mr. Lynda making the acquaintance of another househusband:

"Mr. Lynda and I had decided to meet at a restaurant for supper. He arrived dressed in a nice pair of shorts and a polo shirt. I was late; I had a presentation to make and I was dressed in a dark blue business suit. I ordered for the both of us, unaware that this older man was watching us. He may have been in his early forties. He came up to us before we left and commented on what he had observed. He talked to Mr. Lynda while I paid the bill. He said, 'She has you whipped boy, but there is no better way to be! Just let her have her way. She is going far.' He was on his weekly Boys' Night Out. The other friend he was to meet could not show up at the last minute because one of the children had gotten sick. He has been a househusband for over twenty years. He took Mr. Lynda's number; they are going to get together for a Boys' Night Out until we leave for my job later this summer."

Somewhat kinkier forms of male bonding can take place within the context of FLR couple groups, if the wives are so inclined, as this husband explained in a posting:

"My wife and I recently had a business dinner in which our hosts were another Female Led marriage couple. After many drinks the women encouraged us men to discard our clothing and serve them naked. It was a very powerful first for us and I enjoyed it. It was my first time sharing 'guy' talk and tips with another househubby in a similar situation. The other hubby and I both agreed that sharing our nudity before our fully clothed wives and serving them was truly a powerful reminder of our place in our marriages... It was a thrill to be face-to-face with another submissive househusband."

Another househusband reacted with envy: "You are so lucky! i wish i had the opportunity to talk with someone like myself who has assumed all the traditional duties of the 1950s housewife."

What would two such husbands talk about? According to another posting, a typical interchange might start something like this: "Susannah's husband and I got to talk about being owned and controlled by such wonderful powerful women. How we both realized it was the best way and were glad to have found such loving knowing women to train us properly."

DEGREES (AND DECREES) OF DOMESTICITY

A final word on the topic. from another husband:

"As we move deeper into our FLRs. some of our old lives will recede as our relationship with our Wives becomes our world. Perhaps one way to cope with these painful losses is to forge new friendships with their friends."

Comments:
Bob: I love the part about the husbands who strip in front of their wives and serve them drinks. I think many women would love to relax and talk with their best friend while their husbands wait on them hand and foot.
Mark: Bob. I do enjoy the virtual support group of like-minded wife-led husbands. through message board postings or email exchanges. But it would be very strengthening to be able to enjoy such relationships face to face.

Girls Night Out (10.12.08)

There is. of course. an extra FLR dimension to any discussion of "Boys Night Out." that sacred male-bonding ritual by which some husbands intermittently recreate bachelorhood with the kind of frat-boy behaviors celebrated in beer commercials.

Boys Nights Out can run the gamut from watching an occasional big game with one's buddies at the corner sports bar to cashing out the weekly paycheck at the county-line strip club.

Wife-worshipful husbands. on the other hand. learn to forgo or at least minimize these adolescent excesses. either of their own volition or in compliance with the wishes of their spouses.

All things considered. they much prefer to bond with her.

Some wife-led marriages take things a bit farther. They practice she-he turnabout. where it is the wife who is at liberty to step out on the town with the girls. while hubby stays dutifully behind.

An example would be the FLR union of Nancy and Dennis. chronicled here elsewhere: "Nancy and her friends often have ladies night out." Dennis writes. "where the husbands stay at home with the kids or clean the bathroom."

Do you detect a complaint there? I honestly don't think so. It is, for these made-over males, the new status quo.

Some role-reversing wives actually take their husbands *along* on their girls night out: "Of course," as one such wife explains, "they had to walk behind us and they were not allowed to talk unless we gave them permission."

In the previous post I quoted Au876, describing his disappointment upon learning, at the last minute, that his wife "was going out with a couple of her friends to a movie" and that he should not wait up for her. He promptly began looking for some "surprise chore" to do for her, such as ironing a favorite blouse, while commenting, as if mumbling under his breath: "One thing is for sure, I can't complain to her because that isn't allowed."

At first I thought Au876 was bragging about the obvious inequity of his domestic arrangement, but now I'm wondering if there isn't just the slightest tone of resentment as he reaches for the steam iron. Just wondering, mind you. Certainly there is a tinge of mild protest in this letter to Ken and Emily Addison, co-authors of the provocative "Around Her Finger" books and website materials:

"[My] wife and two girls from her work usually go out one Friday a month. They just go to a local tavern that has a decent happy hour and draws a nice crowd." The husband gives quite a few details before getting around to voicing his complaints about these "girl's nights" after which his wife "almost always comes home much later then she says she will." The husband admits "that jealousy is also a factor here," but eventually talks himself into the idea that what he really needs to do is "to chill out and allow her more freedom."

Ken Addison agrees: "Once you acknowledge that [your wife] is in control and that your first responsibilities are to obey and serve her, you will achieve both a peace of mind and a 'peace of relationship' that is worth many times more than simply getting your way on minuscule points... The next time [your wife] comes home from one of her nights out with the girls, let her know that her new freedom is permanent."

"Social freedom was something I had insisted on even as an undergrad," a young woman attorney writes about her own decidedly wife-led marriage, "but this was generally limited to a girls' night out two or three times each month until my senior year. But once I became a junior law partner and wrested financial control of my marriage, this situation underwent a fundamental change. As a partner in the firm I now had increased social contacts, and hence increased opportunities, with numerous prominent attorneys and clients. The exercise of my social freedom thus increased as a matter of course. In my husband's complete acceptance of my new status, I saw there would never be resistance to me or to my authority."

Some perennially lovestruck husbands even boast about the dramatic disparity between the liberties enjoyed by their wives versus the restrictions placed on themselves: "My wife can go and come as she pleases, do what she wants. She knows I will ask no questions, and while she is gone I will be home either resting or tending my chores awaiting her return. In my book that is the way it should be and she thinks so, too."

Not surprisingly, perhaps, such unequal arrangements can slide into outright cuckoldry, consensual or otherwise. The varying results of these marital and extramarital experiments can be studied in the monthly installments chronicled online by female supremacist Elise Sutton.

Whatever else may be said about cuckoldry, it is risky business, on multiple fronts. Some people like to play with dangerous and combustible materials, others do not. It is decidedly not one of the current or even contemplated steps in turning marriage back into passionate courtship.

At least not in my book.

But a loving and worshipful husband might well enjoy seeing his wife flirt a bit in public, or encourage her to spread her wings socially, to go out more often with her friends, especially girlfriends.

What I have found, in my own marriage, is that my wife comes home after such nights out happier and quite often more amorous. Alcohol may or may not have been poured.

Comments:
Jboy: "Girls Night Out" is an essential ingredient in an WLM. It marks out a Woman's independence and control of the relationship. It gives her the opportunity to enjoy her friends, network with colleagues, hone her social skills and increase her social and business connections. These evenings also allow a Wife to relax a little from her heavy domestic responsibilities as family decision-maker or CEO/CFO and to renew and refresh herself.

The Woman's recreation marks out her hubby as her stay-at-home dependent. Hubby should use the Girl's Night Out as an opportunity to serve his Wife more. He should greet her return lovingly, have the house quiet and neat, prepare a snack or nightcap, listen and let her know how much he missed her. This will make her feel special and adored. When the Wife is out, she will know that she has a loving and obedient hubby at home, missing her and waiting up for her return, eager to lavish on her his love and service.

Mark: That is exactly how it's supposed to work. But even if I haven't gotten my to-do list accomplished when she comes home, and the kids are still wreaking minor havoc, I find she is still appreciative of the time away.

Anonymous: What woman wouldn't want to smugly inform their househusband that she and her friends were going out and that he would be staying home to do housework? His only response could be "Yes, Ma'am."

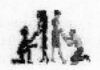

13

SETBACKS AND STEPBACKS

Male Mutiny -- To Quell or Not to Quell (6.25.08)

On a popular FLR message board (she-makes-the-rules.com). there were several postings about husbands rebelling from the FLR status—after having begged for it!

One husband described his occasional bouts of mutinous behavior in this way: "I can become sullen. stubborn. or willful at times due to various reasons. and this causes tension between Goddess and myself."

The responses were thoughtful. insightful. Most of the male posters counseled wives to be understanding and tolerant. Consensus: Adjusting to an FLR and submissive status takes time. no matter what a guy's fantasies have been. and the wife should be understanding of occasional rebellions.

The Case for Zero Tolerance

There is another FLR school of thought. of course. which advises zero tolerance of husbandly mutinies. rebellions. "pissy fits." etc.

The oft-quoted Au876 describes how his wife-leader dealt with him on these occasions:

"I think some form of rebellion is natural no matter how deeply we want to submit. My wife refers to my small rebellions as pouting. She just waits me out and kids me about it. She says

I am pouting or acting like a little boy. She thinks it is funny and childish of me. It may take me a day or two to get over it even though I try hard. When I come around she knows I am just a little more firmly under her control than I was before."

On other occasions, however, Mrs. Au would take a firmer hand with him: "When she senses some rebellion in my attitude or actions she is quick to punish me in some way and warns me I better learn to like things the way they are."

Au876 cites various kinds of punishments, from "writing lines" to a cut in his weekly allowance to a denial of TV or computer time.

A more frightening form of punishment is described by a worshipful husband cyber-tagged "love struck":

"I remember in our early days my Lady responded to a similar situation by taking the initiative and telling me 'OK if that's the way you want it - IT'S OFF!' This worked with me on two levels: 1. I couldn't imagine going back to the way things were before, so I was mortified that I'd pushed her too far. 2. The very act of her taking control in such a dramatic manner revealed an inner strength that immediately increased my desire to serve her. The next day I was begging for her forgiveness. She gave me this and also gave me a very sore bottom to remind me of my place in the relationship."

A philosophical summing up on this topic is offered by Lady Misato of "Real Women Don't Do Housework":

"If resistance is offered at all it will consist merely of token rebellions from time to time for the sake of his ego and to test your resolve and seriousness. In actuality, he will enjoy this as much as you do and he would be extremely disappointed if you were to back away from your new expectations of him."

SETBACKS AND STEPBACKS

Point of No Return (6.13.09)

"Is there a point of no return when one truly embraces this way of life?" "Ms. Kathleen." writing in Elise Sutton's "Predominant" e-magazine. February 2005 issue.

I've noticed a number of female-led relationship blogs bowing out recently. Some go quietly dormant. while others exit with brief regrets on the part of the blogger. almost always male. that there's nothing more to write about. The wife has lost interest in all things FLR. the husband's enthusiasm has consequently faded and fizzled. their relationship has devolved back to the status quo ante.

It's an oft-told tale. Euphoria is a volatile emotion. hard to sustain. There can be a manic quality to the early days of courtship. and of courtship marriages. I'm talking strictly guys now. One week hubby is a passion-primed dynamo. writing love poems and feverish resolutions. buying roses and boxed chocolates. giving footrubs and scrubbing the baseboard. The following week finds him back on the couch. cuddling a remote and frosty lager.

Yet courtship marriages do exist where the initial euphoria lasts long enough to be replaced by a steadier fuel supply. where escape velocity is achieved to a sustainable FLR lifestyle.

As fdhousehusband wrote in his valuable (and sadly discontinued) blog. "To convince my wife that I truly wanted to worship and serve her as my queen took years of dedication to housework. child-rearing and pampering without any thought of reward. I did the chores cheerfully and enthusiastically. Yet. each time I failed and became lazy. I felt that I took several steps backward for both of us. I was moving from one equilibrium to another in terms of our relationship. and I needed to be perfect. not anything in between. not just sometimes. Ultimately I convinced her that this was my life. that I was fulfilled in that role and didn't want anything other than to worship and serve her."

Here is a wife talking about the gradual process of overcoming her own reservations about taking the leading role in her marriage: "It took me a couple of years to really embrace this lifestyle completely. But my husband was incredibly patient with me, offering help when I needed it and backing off when I needed him to. Communication and patience have been the keys for us."

Whether the prime mover is wife or husband, the rule seems to be that progress needs to be gradual and incremental, and both parties need to find real benefits in the altered domestic and romantic arrangements.

There needs to be a comfort level achieved, as well. Courtship marriage, like real successful courtship, has to be anchored in reality and honesty—and in the existing relationship. Wait a minute, I think I may have lifted that last sentence almost intact from an extremely articulate FLR advocate known as "Mistress Rika": "The key to a successful [female-led] relationship is to add the exchange of power to the dynamics of your [existing] relationship rather than to replace existing ones."

But at some point, it seems, there needs to be a milestone, or maybe several such, at which both parties pause and reflect and acknowledge that the experiment is working for both of them. That Fantasyland has morphed into Realityland. That, in a phrase, "There's no going back."

To reach that milestone, Emily and Ken Addisons of the "Around Her Finger" book and blog suggest a one-week FLR boot camp, after which the deal is sealed (or not). The happy AHF boot-campers who report back, not surprisingly, usually have both thumbs-up. "We tried the boot camp about four months ago, and we have never looked back."

Even some initially skeptical wives come out of the boot camp as gung-ho converts to the lifestyle: "Not only did I enjoy my week in charge much more than I imagined that I would, I would never imagine having it any other way. Just as you suggest, I told him in no uncertain terms that from that point on I would expect him to obey me and respect my authority. In the weeks and months that have followed nothing has changed. We have never been happier and I never would have imagined that this would have worked so well."

So, the answer to the question posed at the top of this posting. "Is there a point of no return when one truly embraces this way of life?" is "Yes."

Not always, of course, is the "point of no return" question asked hopefully. Sometimes it is asked with a certain apprehension, even dread, by husbands and boyfriends getting a sudden case of cold feet upon seeing long-cherished fantasies becoming all too real. Just how far down the Female-Led road dare they go before it's too late to turn around and scramble back to "the way things were"?

Like this hapless guy, quoted in Elise Sutton's monthly Q&A column: "I am coming to the realization that I am approaching a point of no return and each step, including reading your book, is taking me there."

Or this guy confessing last-minute FLR jitters: "Is there any chance we could ever go back to being a more traditional husband and wife?"

"The short answer to your question." Ms. Sutton responds. "is No. Why should she and why should you?" Or, as she tells another husband: "[Your wife] may constantly be looking for new activities but I doubt she will ever desire any other type of relationship. She is hooked and she does not want to go back."

Her bottom-line to apprehensive husbands, of course, is a positive pep talk: "Go for it."

Which, I think, is the way most husbands feel upon reaching "the point of no return." These giddy guys, for example:

"It took many years for us to learn how to get along and build a new relationship. I am sure that nobody knows the extent to which she wields the authority in our house now. For what started out as one weekend a month has gradually become second nature 24 7... Like the Nike add says. 'Just Do It.'"

"Having made the choice to live my fantasy, I have never regretted it. Good luck on finding your path."

"My wife's Loving Female Authority over our relationship has gone from habit to lifestyle in just under one year. I would say that we are now firmly embedded in a Female-Led Relationship 24/7. Because of the positive changes in every area of our marriage, we both agree that there is no turning back to our old ways. That door is closed, and the key is gone."

"It would seem that any and all periods of adjustment are over for me, and have been for some time. I feel like I have been reconditioned and have changed so much over the last couple of years, that I am like a different person in so many ways... I arrived at total acceptance."

"Good luck and remember, once you give her all the keys to your heart there is no going back."

"I realized just how pleased and proud I was to be so completely controlled by my wife, how we had already gone beyond a point of no return, and how (deep down) I had always yearned for this ever since we met... It really made me feel in touch with my natural self, and even more accepting of who and what I am."

"My fiancée and I converted to this lifestyle two years ago (at my instigation) and both of us can honestly say that we have never been happier in our lives. Definitely no going back for us! She has adapted to her position of power with far more relish than I ever imagined possible, and our relationship really works."

"Once you get her to accept that part of herself and take charge there is no going back.....but why would you want to? It is so much nicer this way!"

"The female-led lifestyle has changed our lives for the better. We both realize that there is no going back to the way things used to be. We are on a new path now, and we are both giddy about where that path will lead us."

"I can't imagine my wife accepting any laziness from me ever again. I can't imagine her performing sex again as an obligation. I see her thriving in her new role and as much as I love it, it's a bit intimidating. I'm thrilled and terrified... and hope I'm up to the challenges that lay ahead of me."

Any hesitancy on the part of this husband is quickly dismissed by his wife's certainty: "She has come to the point where she feels this is her due, instead of a game we play. Occasionally I have had moments where my interest has flagged, have been too tired from work, etc., but she has shown me that there is no going back, and I love Her so much for this."

Same deal for this husband: "Sometimes I get frightened as to the monumental changes occurring so fast. But obviously there is no going back because my wife has fallen in love with this lifestyle."

And one more: "Once my wife saw all the benefits that were in it for her, she started to get really interested. I've in a sense created a beast and there is no going back."

Female supremacist Paige Harrison apparently dealt with her husband's recalcitrance with a now-hear-this ultimatum: "There will be no going back to how things were before. So I want you to get used to this. This is not a game."

Ditto this take-charge wife, as she confides to Elise Sutton: "My husband and I kept going deeper into FLR and the more we did it, the more I wanted from him. For a while, he was the one who had reservations, and tried to apply the brakes and began to rebel. But eventually he realized there was no stopping me, and that this is no longer a game. This is really our lives and our marriage and there will be no going back."

For one wife, the "point of no return" was before the beginning: "I told my husband that if he wanted me to agree to try this, there would be no going back because I was not going to undertake these big changes only to have him change his mind later."

The opening question of this post was taken from an Elise Sutton's website, and we'll close with a last word of advice from Ms. Sutton to husbands reaching their personal "point of no return":

"You can't go back and you don't want to go back. In fact, you want to go deeper into [this lifestyle]. You want this wonderful woman to take you deeper into submission so that your old life becomes an even more distant memory, so distant that it

229

cannot be seen in the rear-view mirror of your mind."

Comments:

Whatevershesays: Because a consistent wife led marriage evolves, I'm not sure where the point of no return is. This uncertainty is probably compounded by the fits and starts or the 2 steps forward, one step back advancement of a wife led marriage.

Anonymous: I really think I'm just starting to cross this line myself now. It is 2 steps forward and 1 back so often, as WSS said, but my wife appears to be taking to this like a duck to water now. She's not going to want to go back, I can sense that even if she hasn't said it. I can't wait for her to tell me exactly what I already sense is coming. She is and always will be my Queen. PS: Thanks Mark for changing my life with your website and book!

Mark: Maybe WLM's never really leave "2 steps forward, 1 step back" territory, but a lot of forward progress is made this way. So that when I turn around and look way back at the dynamics of our marriage when this all got started, they are very dramatically different—and her power today is increased by leaps and bounds. To prove this, I started making a list of how things are now, areas in which she has asserted or assumed control, or in which I gradually ceded control to her. It's quite a list.

14

HOW AM I DOING, COACH?

Weekend Update, Part 1 (10.24.08)

If you browse the female relationship message boards like "She Makes The Rules" or many others that have come and gone in recent years, or read the monthly Q&As in the "Around Her Finger" blog or on Elise Sutton's Female Superiority site, you'll find a dizzying array of opinions—on financial arrangements, apportioning of household chores, who initiates intimacy, methods of correction, you name it.

On one issue, however, you will find near total agreement—the necessity for continuing communication between both parties to the FLR (female-led relationship) arrangement. Hopes and fears need to be shared, agreements made, goals and timelines set, results evaluated. Or, if that sounds too biz-jargony, let's just say they need to talk. A lot and often.

Emily and Ken Addison of "Around Her Finger" recommend a first foray into a wife-led arrangement be done on a two-week trial, a "boot camp" deal. ("During those two weeks, introduce him to loving female authority as described in the Boot Camp section of the book. At the end of those two weeks, have an open and candid discussion about wife-led marriages...")

Fumika Misato of "Real Women Don't Do Housework" prescribes intimate bedroom "conversations" where the husband, in

231

particular, is encouraged by the wife (and erotically manipulated) into sharing his secret sexual fantasies.

Elise Sutton and others who advocate wife-led or matriarchal marriage recommend husbands keep a journal in which they record their daily thoughts and fantasies for their wives to read. "My wife has me keep a journal which she may read at any time," as one husband explains. "The journal has entries like what she said and how I felt about it."

"All husbands who submit to Loving Female Authority should be required to keep accurate journals," according to one woman who posted under the exalted cybername of "Grand Matriarch." "This will aid them in performing as well as organizing and focusing their attention on their wives. She will then be aware of his mind-set and daily performance of assigned chores, tasks and appointments."

"I have my husband keep a journal and every night at bedtime I go through it with him," agrees another wife. "I want everything in our minds cleared."

Sometimes the journal-reading review is part of a periodic evaluation, in which the wife and husband discuss progress in their FLR, or the lack of it, or share their thoughts on the process.

This seems most frequently to be conducted on a weekly basis (often on Sunday evenings) and is variously described as an "assessment," or a "performance evaluation" or "performance review," and, in one instance, even as a "weekly update."

In cases where the wife has assumed control of family finances, the "weekly update" may be combined with the awarding of the husband's weekly allowance. Other agenda items may include a discussion of weekly menus (for husbands who cook), or measuring progress toward an agreed-upon goal (like for husbands trying to shed pounds).

And, of course, there are wives for whom the weekly performance review is the time to assess and mete out appropriate punishments for their partners' shortcomings over the week past.

In many cases, the weekly review is a give-and-take discussion. in which husbands and wives share their concerns and work to reach consensus for proceeding. This is certainly the case when a couple meets to evaluate a trial FLR arrangement. such as the two-week boot camp mentioned above. But. judging by my online research. the longer the female-led dynamic endures. the more likely the weekly conference will evolve. by mutual consent. into a courtroom with the wife as judge and the husband as judgee.

It's the Lady of the House who keeps score. in other words. And it may not be enough that hapless hubby complete his weekly honey-do list. There may be other columns in the evaluation sheet. How well did he do his assigned tasks? Did he complain? Second guess her? Talk back? Sulk? Delay? Forget things?

Is this an unfair and one-sided tribunal? Of course. But almost without exception. the wife-worshipping husbands who share their experiences online indicate that they want their wives to keep score. to evaluate them. to give them feedback. and even to use training or discipline to improve their performance.

As one guy put it: "I think this is a great idea for all husbands. We need to know where we stand. what we do well. and where we need improvements."

To illustrate (and bolster) the point. let me offer additional examples:

"My new routine this year includes a weekly evaluation of my performance by my Wife on Sunday evening. She gave me praise during Her January 6th review; January 13th was a different matter..."

This husband goes on to relate how he received several demerits for not completing all his chores to her satisfaction in a timely fashion. But this was not the worst. His wife had discovered a speeding ticket he had failed to tell her about. His subsequent punishment (which I will not get into) was as much for the attempted coverup as for the actual offense.

Are such evaluations always negative? Apparently not. On a subsequent session. this husband boasts that "my Wife was so pleased with my progress that She awarded me two additional hours to play on the computer."

Another husband writes: "My wife seemed pleased with my weekly work performance, although I was chastised for forgetting a few personal tasks she told me to do. Like yesterday, I was supposed to pick up her dress at the cleaners, but I forgot."

There is a persuasive tone of sincerity in the accounts of these wife-following husbands. They really do want to learn to better serve their wonderful wives in as many ways as possible.

Hence, one devoted husband proposed to his wife that she evaluate his performance in much the same manner that she did her subordinates on her executive-level job. "That's a good idea for you," was her enthusiastic comeback. "I'll come up with a form that YOU will fill out, then I will then critique your self-evaluation and we will institute some additional training to get you where I think you should be."

Lady Misato also thinks this is a good idea: "The mere act of keeping track of his behavior will have a profound effect on your husband. Not only is his every behavior subject to an indelible record avoiding any possibility that you might forget either the act or your feelings about it, but in addition the constant state of evaluation will elevate your power over him and further invite his surrender to your will."

"The first step," she continues, "is, of course, to keep track. Make a habit of keeping a notepad handy at all times either in your purse or in a pocket. The idea is to record your reaction to your husband's behavior at the instant of the behavior. If you trust your memory of if you simply do not enjoy keeping track throughout the day, you can simply make a mental review of the day each night."

A semi-serious (and discontinued) online femdom magazine calling itself "Whap!" came up with a playful take on this weekly-wifely checkup:

"Setting aside one night at week's end is the easiest way to monitor and correct your husband's behavior before things get out of hand. I recommend that you make it a weekly ritual in your house. The procedure is simple. Make sure all your husband's weekly chores are done. including cleaning. laundry and kitchen duties. Are your shoes polished and in order? Your bras and panties laundered and put away? Your vanity table organized? Your jewelry cleaned and polished? Is his housework up to your high standards? Were the meals he prepared creative and delicious or just thrown together? What about errands—did he pick up your dry cleaning. do the food shopping and remember what brand of tampons to buy? Finally. did he take it upon himself to do any special projects? Don't overlook anything."

The tone here. of course. is unmistakably tongue-in-cheek. but. in plain fact. for many couples this kind of itemized weekly accounting is routine reality.

"We have established tasks (chores & attitude adjustments for me) and a weekly review session similar to normal work evaluation reports." a husband explains matter-of-factly. "I know in my heart we must agree to some penalties if I am to have any success complying with her directions and reaching the performance goals we agree upon."

Another husband and wife codified the agenda of their weekly meeting into formal contractual language:

"Performance will be assessed once a week. normally Monday afternoon. Linda will review John's goals and comment on his performance for the week. John will be given a chance to explain any transgressions and should take this time to confess anything that has not been discussed. At Linda's discretion. John may be given correction via discipline so that his performance will improve."

What other provocative little domestic rituals are observed during these weekly updates? I'll save them for Part 2 of this double posting.

Comments:
Cuckold and Mistress: We have found journal writing as suggested in this post to be extremely valuable and imagine that a female dominated marriage would be immeasurably harder without it.
Mark: I'm like other guys in not-so-advanced FLRs: my medium-of-

choice for confessing my thoughts to my wife is email. I envy you. How exciting on a daily basis, or wherever, to have her looking over your shoulder, as it were, into your heart and soul and mind.

Weekend Update, Part 2 (10.27.08)

In many wife-led households, the weekly performance review (as discussed in the previous post) has a strong financial component.

The husband may turn over his weekly pay envelope (if it isn't direct-deposited electronically into his wife's account) along with receipts for every dollar spent in the past seven days—as prelude and prerequisite to his wife handing him his adjusted allowance for the week ahead.

But pocket money is certainly not the only thing a man may receive from his wife's hand on such ritual occasions:

"When we first began our relationship," one husband writes, "my wife kept a notebook in which she would record my infractions (not listening, giving her back-talk, not doing something to her specifications), and then she would administer a weekly correction, meting out whatever she decided for each bad behavior."

Or, as described from the distaff side, "Each Sunday evening, I review my husband's performance from the previous week and determine if punishment or reward is required."

I carefully avoided certain "trigger" terms and concepts in my book, *Worshipping Your Wife*. Since the emphasis was on romantic courtship, I didn't want to scare off potential readers with images that could conjure up strange rituals of domestic "punishment" and "discipline."

Which is why I, with many others, have welcomed the much-needed rebranding of this lifestyle under more mainstream banners—e.g., "Loving Female Authority," "Female Led Relationships" and "Wife Led Marriages."

HOW AM I DOING. COACH?

All the same. "corrective measures" such as spanking and paddling are indeed employed by some couples who practice Loving Female Authority. *et al.* For example:

"My wife grades my weekly performance in my domestic chores as well as my sexual service of her. If I do not excel in her opinion. I may receive a painful encouragement with her hairbrush."

Other wives prefer to correct their mates' misbehavior with lighter methods—a stern look. an occasional scolding.

At the weekly reminder session other wives employ school-marmish methods. such as assigning corner time or having the husband write lines. or denying or limiting certain masculine privileges. such as watching the next Big Game or nights out with the boys (see my post on this).

One wife prefers to give her husband an occasional light tap on the top of his head with a rolling pin. It's a most effective and economical reminder. he reports.

And what about rewards? A reinstatement of privileges is one easy option. but the reward of choice for many husbands is simply being granted "release." And no. I'm not talking about a furlough.

"My wife and I are considering a point system where I am awarded points for completing weekly/monthly tasks (cleaning. taking the trash out. things like that). I must earn a minimum of 150 points before she'll even consider allowing me sexual release. Getting the 150 points isn't easy—but worth the effort."

"If the score is sufficient then release is granted." Fumika Misato explains this kind of system. where the husband is kept in wife-supervised chastity. "Otherwise not. Again. you wipe the slate and start over for the next period. In addition. you can vary his allowance and other privileges according to his score. Excel is a great tool for recording and computing scores."

Another reward husbands may enjoy at a weekly assessment is an opportunity to speak more freely about any reservations or complaints they may harbor about domestic arrangements.

"It is my husband's safety valve." one wife explains. "as the rest of the time we have agreed that he is not to question or raise doubts about my control of things. During our weekly sessions, I of course acknowledge whatever my husband says, but he understands that I am under no pressure to act upon any of the requests he makes."

"[These] weekly sessions," according to Elise Sutton, "will ensure the power exchange and the power dynamics of the female-led relationship, motivating [the husband] for the week ahead."

"My wife never raises her voice at our Friday weekly review," explains another worshipful husband, "but simply, in normal conversation tone, admonishes in a way that can strike fear and sadness into me, if I've fallen short in some way. Fear, because I know there will be a punishment coming, and sadness because I have disappointed her in some specific way. When she has finished her lecture, she always asks if I fully understand."

One husband found himself under his wife's scrutiny around the clock. She had been his colleague at work—until she was promoted to head of his department. Suddenly he was having his performance reviewed by her both at home and on the job—with the latter being the more embarrassing: "It humiliated me to have to go once a week to her office and report on my weekly activities, with her sitting in her leather armchair, while I had to sit on a simple chair. It made me feel naked and impotent."

Of course, he wasn't actually naked seated before his wife-boss at work, but he may well have been when being reviewed by her at home. A naked and even kneeling husband is a common ritual aspect in many of these weekly conferences. For instance:

"I will order [my husband] to undress and kneel before me. At that time, I will begin to critique his weekly performance of his chores. I will scold him if he disobeyed me during the week or displayed a negative attitude. I speak in soft whispers, challenging him to be a better husband and informing him of my demands for the week ahead. He yields to my quiet authority and surrenders his will over to me. This brings peace to my husband

and love and harmony to our marriage. In fact. our little sessions usually lead to a night of passion and sex."

But even kneeling is not enough for this hubbie: "On Sunday evenings I lie at [my wife's] feet while she reviews my perform-ance. making notes on the calendar to track my performance over time. At the end of our meeting. she assigns projects for the following week. determines and administers punishment. This system doesn't take much of her time to manage yet effectively satisfies our respective needs."

"We discuss my husband's performance and other things dur-ing those conversations." a wife comments in recommending the practice to other couples. "We have been doing this for several years and find the time very enjoyable."

Here's a husband who certainly seems to enjoy being "dressed down" by his wife (perhaps after being "undressed" by her): "Our weekly conversation was focused on my perform-ance. She evaluated me in several areas. sexual and non-sexual. It was delightful and it turned me on to be taking a very honest look at my good points and bad points."

A final quote illustrates how a weekly tête-a-tête can look be-yond the husband's behavior-of-the-week to take stock of the overall progress of the female-led aspect of the relationship:

"The other night." a husband writes. "we were talking about the changes that we've seen in our relationship. and she said. 'If I've changed you this much in a couple of years. imagine what it will be like in another 10 or 20!' It's a thought that's exciting. but not without a bit of apprehension."

Ready for your gold stars and demerits. guys?

Comments:
Anonymous: I really like the idea of a weekly review report and am wondering if you or others out there would like to share theirs? I have one myself I'm working on and am happy to forward on.

Mark: I'd very much like to see the weekly review report that you are de-veloping. And I'd like it even more if I could get my wife to inaugurate this kind of weekly ritual with me—not that she doesn't point out things I haven't done or mistakes I've made.

Anonymous: Last night I showed my wife the categories of performance.

such as domestic support, and she set scoring criteria for each. The ratings were: excellent, satisfactory, needs improvement, and unacceptable. After she specified what I had to do to meet her expectations, she rated my performance. I got an unacceptable in 'companionship'—have to do better at going on walks with her. This is all new to me, but I'm really happy with the way she's helping me.

A Clean Slate (11.11.08)

This is just a postscript to my two-part "Weekend Update" postings. In a recent collection of "Real Life Stories" on Elise Sutton's site, "Doreen B" writes about the weekly performance review that she administers to her live-in lover, Timothy, 20 years her junior:

"Each week I appraise his efforts for the week just gone by and explain to him where I require improvement or more effort. I then decide whether he deserves punishment (he always does!) and inform him of how many strokes with my strap or cane and/or extra days in his device that I have decided to award him."

This is standard operating procedure in female-led relationships." But then "Doreen" cites an additional benefit of these sessions, which I thought merited a mention here:

"…the weekly appraisal has become an important part of our relationship. It lays down the standards I expect and closes off one week and starts a new one with a clean sheet. Timothy says this is particularly important for him, as he feels cleansed and forgiven for any mistakes or faults and able to concentrate on getting things right for the coming week."

This recurring rite of passage has the effect of wiping the husband's slate clean and re-energizing and rededicating him for the coming week's service to his beloved.

"When I am finished," she adds, "[Timothy] kneels at my feet

and thanks me for correcting him and promises to work even
harder for me in the future."

Comments:
Anonymous: Lucky man!

Mark: Anonymous. I join you in that envious ejaculation. My shortcomings just accumulate. and there seems no mechanism for cleaning the slate or
expiating them. Perhaps an occasional confessional would not offend her sen-
sibilities?

15

BEHIND CLOSED DOORS

Whispering the "P" Word, Part 1 (9.1.09)

In "Worshipping Your Wife," both book and blog, I have tiptoed around the theory and practice of punishment in female-led relationships. I've touched on it in this blog, but you can search the book in vain for the word "discipline" or "spanking" or "punishment."

My purpose, as I've explained, has been to emphasize the romantic, courtship nature of female- and wife-led relationships and loving female authority.

This is the appeal that I made initially, and continue to make, to my own wife in regard to this lifestyle, ignoring any practices that might put her off. Like spanking or paddling hubby, standing him in the corner, and so forth. (I'll fill in some of the blanks lower down.)

And yet, the "P" word won't go away. Clearly, "Loving Female Authority" presumes a Loving Female vested with the Authority to enforce her will on her guy. Likewise, a Female- or Wife-Led relationship requires a male who follows the woman's lead. As in any leadership structure, there must be incentives for good performance and disincentives for poor performance, for not following directives. And, in an FLR, it is she who must be empowered to administer those "disincentives," i.e., penalties or punishments.

So, despite all previous resolutions, I am going to devote the next several postings here to an informal survey of some penalties and punishments currently employed to guide and enhance female-led coupling. FLR message boards are teeming with examples, of course, but I'm going to steer well clear of the kinkier sort, in favor of those trending more to the playful and provocative.

For example, as befits Lady Misato's paradigm of knightly courtship, picture a brawny knight, stripped of his armor for whatever infraction or shortcoming, being toyed with by a delicate damsel, no longer distressed but perhaps doing a bit of the distressing.

I'm going to let others do most of the talking, as my own wife does not paddle or punish me physically. Indeed, it is hard to imagine her doing this (although, believe me, I've tried). She explained her reluctance this way, after one of my abject failures to carry out her wishes: "You're an adult, and I won't punish you." (You'll find more about this objection to disciplining the adult male later on in this series of postings.)

But I did not get off scot-free. My wife expressed her disappointment with me very clearly at that time, and I felt it keenly, as I was meant to. She consigned me to the doghouse, just not literally. Such wifely disapproval, as any husband can attest, can be very powerful, all the more so because it just seethes and simmers for excruciating hours without boiling over.

And my wife's full-spectrum emotions *are* powerful. Positive or negative, they permeate the entire household, me and the kids. I am helplessly attuned to whatever vibe she is putting out.

As the old saying goes, "When Mama ain't happy, ain't nobody happy!" And right here is the first good argument to be made for the "P" word, or maybe "CP"—corporal punishment within the safe and consensual framework of a female-led relationship: A paddling allows angry wife and errant hubby a convenient catharsis, an intimate and effective ritual for remorse and reorientation.

This husband, a long-standing member of the self-explanatory Disciplinary Wives Club, puts it more plainly: "We have never gone to bed mad. My wife knows that I have paid for anything I have done that displeases her or for having a generally bad attitude."

Another husband offers a similar salute to his own wife's strong right arm: "You must admit that her method for settling arguments, spanking, was much better than getting the cold treatment for days."

Lady Misato, creator of "Real Women Don't Do Housework," states the case with eloquent and elegant simplicity:

"One of the advantages of female-led relationships over conventional relationships, [an advantage] which promotes harmony and ends hostilities, is that they have an additional tool for solving disputes, which has to do with penance. Instead of storing up resentments and dissatisfactions, the wife is allowed to discharge them by imposing penance."

Misato continues, addressing wives and compressing an entire essay into two sentences: "Penance provides you with a means to overcome your anger, pain, and frustration at your husband. Penance provides your husband with an opportunity to express his love and remorse by enduring the punishment you have selected."

In the same vein, Loving Female Authoritarian Elise Sutton instructs a husband that he should be grateful to his wife for taking appropriate corrective measures: "Your wife is a wise woman. She is using her feminine power to bring peace and harmony to your marriage and she is defusing arguments."

Such corrective measures, Misato points out, need not be restricted to physical punishment or discipline:

"Ideally, you should always have a punishment available for any given wrong. Thus there is always a means for restoring the marriage to a state of mutual respect and love. Indeed, a husband's transgressions become an opportunity to have some great fun. In practice you may find that there are some wrongs that are not so easily set right and which try your patience."

Among the penalties Misato suggests are "extra chores. either constructive. like washing your car. or valueless. like writing sentences."

A great many wives prefer to correct their husbands shortcomings with such alternate means—a stern look. a weekly reminder session or evaluation. a quick scolding. Others prefer schoolmarmish remedies such as assigning corner time. the writing of repetitive lines. or denial of certain privileges. such as watching sports or going out with the boys or computer time. One wife prefers to give her husband a sharp thwack on the top of his head. He knows what it means.

Exile from milady's bed or bedchamber is another frequent chastisement. a variation of the doghouse. As this husband comments: "I find that sleeping on the floor next to her is very humbling and help keeps me in the proper frame of mind."

A wife adds: "I have used it as a punishment on several occasions in the past. I allow him a 2-inch thick foam pad and a blanket. As for the kids. daddy has a sore back and sleeping on the mat helps it feel better."

Writing lines is a very effective method. according to the oft-quoted Au876. Once. on a trip. Au was forced to stay up all night in a motel lobby writing lines after he had neglected to bring along his wife's favorite toenail polish. I kid you not.

In the morning. after his hand-cramping all-nighter. he took the stack of papers along with some coffee to her bedside: "She asked if I got any sleep—no. Were my hands tired—very. Should she count the sentences—no. I had numbered them for her. She took the stack of papers and thumbed through them. She asked if I thought I would ever forget her polish again. I haven't and I won't. She has used the same type punishment several times since. It is very effective. takes none of her time and I assure you it works."

Washing hubby's mouth out with soap for bad language or talking back also smacks of the schoolmistress. of course. and works. A recent example appeared on the She Makes The Rules message board, concerning a husband who used profanity in front of a neighbor. He detailed the immediate and humiliating consequences: "My wife not only washed my mouth out with a softened bar of clear soap but afterward marched over to the woman's place, made me apologize, and offer to make amends."

The husband complained about what he considered his wife's unfairness—imposing a lot of extra chores—but got zero sympathy from other posters on the female-led message board: "Show your wife - and the neighbour - this post of yours," one husband shot back. "Bet you will get another dose of discipline and it will be deserved! Be grateful for the discipline you get and don't whine."

"Admit you made a mistake," advised another. "Take your punishment. Tell them both how really sorry you are. And don't repeat the behavior."

A no-nonsense wife provided the summing-up: "One of my standard lines that I am sure my husband gets sick of hearing is, 'You wanted a wife led marriage and now you have one!' I think that is the biggest problem - making the man see that this is now what life is. Take your punishment and be thankful it's not worse."

"Minor offences are handled with a loss of privileges," another wife confides. "My husband is a huge sports fan. You name it and he watches it or plays it. If he does not do his chores on schedule or does them poorly, he is not allowed to watch TV. If it happens more than once or twice in a week, he will lose tennis or golf with his buddies. No exceptions are allowed."

All very effective penalties, none requiring the wife to lay a finger on her guy. But what about the wifely right to bear arms? Or bare arms? I'll delve more deeply in the next posting on this topic.

End Part 1

Comments:

WSS: My wife doesn't punish. Occasionally she'll deny me sex or make me sleep on the floor but it's so infrequent that it's hardly worth mentioning. Perhaps I'm just too good to be punished? LOL NOT.

Anonymous: I do punish my husband, but it is very seldom. He has become so good in the past several years we have been practicing our wife led relationship that there is not much need for it. But he will displease me every so often, not on purpose but just forgetting who is in charge or not doing his housework perfectly.

I think this is a good topic to write about and ask for comments since all wife led relationships involve some form of punishment, even if it's the silent treatment, extra chores, or a sit down session once a week to go over what was done wrong, and what was done right. I will be sitting down with my husband every Friday night and will review the last seven days. This way he will be off to a good start for the weekend.

He Is Mine All Mine: I agree with the prior post, in WLR there is always some form of punishment administered to errant husbands. Just showing anger towards him and making him feel that he was totally wrong (which husbands always are, never wives), giving him the doghouse treatment, or making him come around to beg for your forgiveness (buying you flowers or a make up gift), are all forms of punishments. They don't have to be about spanking him.

Worshipped By Him: I think the best punishment for any husband is restricting their orgasms when they displease their wife, or if they didn't do a proper job on their housework. My husband must wait 4 weeks for an orgasm, and weeks (or I have threatened months) are added for *any* bad behavior. Ladies, this is the easiest punishment you can administer to your husband, you don't have to lift a finger, just make him wait longer. Plus you get the added benefit of having him stay horny longer, the hornier he gets, the more he will try to please you.

Whispering the 'P' Word, Part 2 (9.12.09)

The preceding post surveyed various methods of "Punishment Lite"—none requiring the wife to lay a finger on her guy. "But what," I asked in closing, "about the wifely right to bear arms?"

In wife-led marriages, some wives emphatically do (use corporal punishment), a lot or a little, some wives don't at all, some are averse, some squeamish, some just a wee bit curious about it. I'll include a few quotes from across that spectrum, from both wives and husbands.

Rationale for Reluctant-to-Punish Wives

Here are a few provocative exchanges between two wives, the first curious but hesitant, the second a confirmed believer in not sparing the rod. They are excerpted (with cyber-names removed) from the original Venus on Top Yahoo forum (precursor to the She Makes The Rules message board).

First Wife: "Recently he has been getting disobedient as if he is testing me and wants me to punish him... I have wondered if spanking might be an option worth trying? I'm not sure I could hurt him though... I believe having it as a threat rather than a regular thing would be enough after having done it once. Maybe also occasionally to show him who is in charge."

Second Wife: "The major obstacle in my mind [to using corporal punishment] wasn't a fear of hurting him so much as a reluctance to treat my husband like a child. (After all, I already have four children. I don't want to raise my husband. I want him to be my partner.) However, I now consider it an invaluable tool in our FLR. I now use spanking not as a means of 'teaching' my husband so much as I do a means of expressing my own displeasure. When he steps out of line, he knows there is a price to pay and, consequently, thinks twice about his behavior. Spanking has produced wonderful results for us over the years."

(Several days later)

First Wife (thanking Second Wife for her advice and encouragement): "I never in my wildest dreams thought I would be doing this [spanking] but I'm OK with it if it helps our relationship. He needs this. It feels strange at the moment but I'm sure I will get used to it."

Second Wife: "I am so delighted that you have come to terms with the idea of correcting his behaviour. I fully appreciate that punishment is not part of everyone's relationship. However, where he feels that it is needed and you are comfortable with using it in order to correct behaviour. I think it can increase the bond between you. You are telling him how important he is to you. After all, you love him, your husband, enough to use a tool he wishes you to use to make him the person you want. He wants to be a better person for you and you are helping him. When he has behaved badly, you have not simply turned away from him in disappointment, you have engaged with him to make him better.

"You are discovering the joys of having your needs/wishes/ views respected and satisfied. Consider that both you and your husband have agreed that these will be respected and satisfied and you are simply helping both of you achieve what you both want.

"Yes, it can be hard work but I find using my hand and alternating with something else can ease the work. And doing it more often can ease any physical tension you feel and help you build up a steady rhythm. However you decide to punish him, make sure he fully understands what he did wrong and how you feel about his disobedience and why you want to punish him in this way."

Punishment as Catharsis
This has already been touched on. But, as is often the case, I think Fumika Misato makes the point most succinctly:

"Spanking can be very cathartic for both parties. Men are particularly fond of enduring physical pain in their devotion to love or in the service of an important cause. For men enduring physical pain can be a powerful symbol of manhood. All the more when that pain is at the request of their love."

This husband seems wholeheartedly in accord: "What I find very hard is the grumpy not-talking-to you punishment. I would rather corporal punishment over that anytime, especially if it came with verbalization of the issue."

"A prompt hard spanking can help restore harmony," another husband remarks: "Reducing her husband to a sincerely remorseful, tearful boy is cathartic for her and, I believe, tends to bring out her natural maternal instincts. By that I mean, her tendency to want to forgive and express her love. 'Honey, I had to punish you because of your behavior, not because I don't love you. I'll always love you, but I'll always correct you for misbehavior.'

"Her nurturing side comes out and this is satisfying for her. For the husband, he has 'paid the price' in a very obvious way. The price that has been determined by his wife as the cost of her forgiveness. He is off the hook as far as guilt goes which, at least to me and I'm sure many others, is extremely important. He should cry tears not only of pain but of emotional release. For the spanking to be truly cathartic, I believe those tears are necessary."

From another husband: "My Princess spanks me when she feels it is necessary but it is very much a last resort after everything else has failed. I know I have upset her deeply when she says I am to be spanked and I take the punishment gladly because I know I deserve it and I feel terrible for disappointing her. Neither of us enjoys it but it draws a line under my disrespectful behavior and enables me to then refocus on pleasing her and making up for my misdemeanors. Afterwards we reaffirm our love for each other and move on."

Which draws this approving feminine response: "I like particularly the point about it drawing a line under the matter. I think it is so much better than nagging. The matter is over, done, dealt with and the parties move on. As you say, afterwards you reaffirm your love for each other. For me spanking is all about restoring the balance in a FLR. If I am offended, upset, I need something that will reconcile me to my partner. I do not want to carry around my annoyance because I believe that this could mar the relationship."

As parting shots on catharsis, let's hear from two husbands, one who gets spanked, and one who only wishes he did:

Gets Punished: "My wife punishes me when I have done a stupid thing and when the punishment is over she feels better and there the anger or grudge is over."

Only Wishes He Did: "There have been times when I wished she would just spank me to get it out of her system. And there have been times when I almost said that to her."

Punishment as Attitude Adjustment

Confession: I'm a typical won't ask for directions guy, often refusing even when I'm obviously lost and directly ordered to do so by my exasperated wife. I find it easier to simply drive around endlessly, hoping to blunder into the right way.

One wife, driven far beyond exasperation when her husband refused to stop at any number of motels, finally ordered him to pull off the road, took the wheel and stopped at the next lighted motel. Then...

"Once in our room, I lit into him and gave him a darn good spanking, surprising him and myself. I felt that he hadn't been listening and in refusing to stop, made for an unsafe and scary drive. Since then, I have a small flogger keychain in the car's glove box, and he knows when I take it out, that I'm putting him on notice about his driving habits."

For an apparently growing cohort of in-charge wives, spanking is the quickest way to take hubby outside of his self-controlled comfort zone and make him think about things. Many other wives, of course, balk at the notion of putting palm or paddle to hubby's nether regions.

How to cure such wifely squeamishness? The advice of a female supremacist calling herself Litia is short and to the point: "Oh my God, just spank him! The wives who say they will never do that always end up eating their words after the 14th time they're getting ready for bed and the dinner dishes aren't done. When you start to see or hear him slack off and you begin to do his chores, sooner or later it will come to you that all who came before you as women of loving authority knew what they were talking about. Spare the rod and you spoil it all."

For a militant minority of female authoritarians, the instrument of choice for attitude adjustment is not the hairbrush or paddle, but the whip. The mere threat of this fearsome punishment is usually sufficient to correct any recalcitrant husband, for example:

"Last night, we took a long walk to the grocery store instead of driving and my wife told me that she did not like my attitude and if I did not change it right now, she would adjust it with the whip when we got home. I reevaluated my attitude right then. I *know* she would carry through on her threat and we are not talking about a sensual whipping."

Another word for attitude adjustment is "training." Hence, on many female-led websites you will see links to various books about how animal training techniques can be successfully employed on husbands and boyfriends. No-nonsense titles like these:

How to Make Your Man Behave in 21 Days or Less Using the Secrets of Professional Dog Trainers by Karen Salmansohn

The Boyfriend Training Kit by Tanya Sassoon

Husband-ry 101, How to Train Your Husband to Be the Spouse You've Always Wanted Him to Be by Michael H. McCann

The sagacious and savvy Fumika Misato goes into considerable depth on behavioral or operant conditioning of the male on her seminal website, "Real Women Don't Do Housework."

Does this sort of wife-administered Pavlovian regimen work? You darn betcha, at least according to this guy: "It is strange that, while I don't really want the corporal punishment my wife delivers, at the same time I can't think of a better feedback mechanism to improve my general behavior and performance of my duties."

This, of course, links back to the topic of weekly performance evaluations, covered in an earlier two-part posting, "Weekend Update."

Punishment as Revenge (and Therapy)

Every now and again, as you explore the online resources about loving female authority in all its manifestations, you will come across another category of female-to-male punishment. These are punishments administered by women, often strong feminists, as a kind of therapeutic "revenge by proxy"—using a boyfriend or husband, who may be faultless, as a kind of whipping boy or stand-in for the entire male population for years, decades, centuries or millennia of perceived masculine or patriarchal sins, i.e., "sins of the fathers."

Elise Sutton, while condoning this kind of vicarious exercise, does suggests that it does not meet the standards of Loving Female Authority:

"Once you enter into a relationship with a man that you care for, discipline and corporal punishment will become less about taking revenge on the male gender who mistreated you and more about loving female authority... That is not to say that you still cannot express your aggressive side and take out some of life's frustrations as you dominate the man you love, but it will take on a different dynamic... You may desire that the man you love stand in proxy for other men who have mistreated you, but your love and compassion as a woman will temper your discipline as you combine strict discipline with nurturing."

Have I exhausted the no-longer-verboten topic? Not quite. I have just enough for one more posting.

Comments:

Anonymous: While I find the idea of LFA intriguing, I balk at the idea of corporal punishment against husbands for the same reason that I balk at male supremacists within certain Judeo-Christian or Islamic communities using that same practice against women.

But if two consenting adults enjoy it and find that it enhances their relationship, that's cool with me. As a straight-up, fair-is-fair feminist type, though, I probably wouldn't be able to do it. Then again, I wouldn't have really gone for LFA at all if my boyfriend hadn't pointed me in the direction of your blog, the Addisons' and Lady Misato's.

I'm still new to all this stuff, but I must say that your blog has made the LFA philosophy seem really appealing, and relatable to the average Joe (or Jane). Even as a so-called liberal grad student of the Y-generation, I have to admit that some of the heavier stuff has squicked me out.

Mark: My wife would agree with you, which is why I've avoided the topic pretty much till now. I decided to go ahead, and was interested in some of the rationales for punishment that I presented. But my own wife chooses not to coerce my compliance or follow-through on what I've promised or she has "asked" me to do. It's up to me to follow if I truly want to honor her as my leader, and I do, so I do.

Anonymous: I can't imagine how difficult LFA is to sustain in marriage. My boyfriend and I have only been practicing it for six months... He gave me your book along with the Addisons', and yours was the one that really sold me on the idea. It's certainly a great alternative to Dr. Laura.

Anonymous: I, too, don't spank my husband. I raised 2 children and am not looking to raise a third. But I will not allow him to get off with nothing after he does something that I don't like. I feel it's better to make him do plenty of housework instead of standing him in a corner for several hours. Also, I do agree that the best punishment is not letting your husband have an orgasm for maybe four to eight weeks, depending what he did.

Rex: My wife is [also] unwilling to use corporal punishment... Corporal punishment would be an overt validation of our WLM. I try to live by the precepts of wife worship for its own sake but without any feedback from my wife I am too often subject to my fickle will.

Mark: Rex, may I suggest you start a list of "half-full" accomplishments in your Wife-Led Marriage so far, rather than fixing too much on the "half-empty" part of the glass? You may, as I was, be surprised and encouraged as to how far you've traveled down this rewarding path.

Whispering the 'P' Word, Part 3 (10.3.09)

As promised, I have just enough for a final posting on the hot-button topic of punishment within a wife-led marriage. I begin with what many wives consider the bottom-line rationale for taking hubby in tow, from time to time:

Punishment as Reminder

Some wife-administered punishments, whether gentle or firm, are designed to remind the male, from time to time or perhaps on a daily basis, of his subordinate position in the relationship, and the power imbalance in favor of the woman.

Sometimes it's just a reminder that there is an agreement in place, a female-led arrangement, and that there are consequences for failure to comply with that agreement. To wit:

"I knew that my husband would need frequent reminders of his new role in our house. The hairbrush merely reinforces my rule as the head of our household."

Such a reminder session is not intended to be erotic. Indeed, it can become tedious, as FLR couples counselor Paige Harrison explains: "I do believe in discipline and I use a variety of disciplinary techniques to remind my husband of who is in charge. This is important. But what you also must recognize is that a disciplinary approach can become tedious and for some women it is just not fun."

Tedious but necessary, according to this husband whose spouse is a member in good standing of the Disciplinary Wives Club: "My wife feels that if I have not received a sound spanking for a couple of weeks, I need a reminder of who sets the rules."

One husband receives such a "reminder" as a wake-up call every morning when he and his wife are traveling—"because my mood changes and I am not as attentive to her when we travel. I may be looking around, etc., and not helping the way I should." The morning session "solves that problem," he adds. "All I can say is it works."

Another husband holds identical views: "Corporal punishment on a regular basis does wonders for our communication & makes me more attentive to her & helps keep me focused on her. She keeps me in line & my life is one of total devotion & service to her."

Might such testimonials from spanked husbands persuade a few reluctant wives to roll up their sleeves and roll down hubby's trousers?

This wife certainly believes in a hands-on solution to marital management: "I am firmly of the opinion that a male with a perpetually sore bottom has a constant reminder of the need to always do his best."

Obviously, while wife-imposed, even this form of not-so-gentle reminder is administered by prior agreement of both parties, Mrs. and Mr. And often, it is the husband who has recognized the need for periodic no-nonsense reminders. I'll start with VeezKnight, who blogs insightfully at "Wife-Led Marriage":

"Most, if not all, submissive men need and want to be disciplined. This is to say they want to be physically reminded of their submissive role in the relationship. The reminders may or may not involve the infliction of pain, but for some reason, a man generally enjoys enduring physical pain at the hand of a woman he loves."

This husband goes even farther, from endurance to apparent enjoyment of harsh wifely reminders: "The marks I carry today are priceless reminders of my love for her and my dedication to her. Plus, I find carrying such reminders around to be very erotic."

Reminder spanking are sometimes referred to as "maintenance spankings," as this wife explains: "Personally, I think that a 'maintenance spanking' can, for some relationships, be as beneficial as orgasm control. In such cases no punishment need to have been earned."

The practice is fairly widespread among female led relationships, at least judging by the candid testimony of these next husbands:

"My weekly behavior is reviewed regularly each week, usually on Saturday mornings. If my behavior has been acceptable for the past week, I am given just a reminder spanking of between five and twenty-five swats with the paddle as a reminder of who is the boss and to behave for the coming week. This has worked very effectively for us."

"I do get a weekly maintenance spanking and punishment spankings whenever my wife feels I need it. I love her very much and wouldn't have it any other way now. I don't always think that way during the spanking, but after it's over and I do my corner time. I give my wife a hug and tell her how much I love her."

"My wife can sense when my behavior is gradually getting less satisfactory. So she takes preventive measures. She calls those non-punishment sessions 'maintenance spankings.' and for me it really works."

"After several years now. I am very obedient and compliant. do all my chores on time and to my wife's satisfaction. Therefore. I rarely merit actual punishment. Instead. I receive regular maintenance training with whatever instrument she chooses. Afterward. I feel cleansed and refreshed so that that I can continue to serves my wonderful lady wife."

"I envision a maintenance spanking as a ritual that allows your wife to express any built-up frustration at you that she may have been hiding so you can learn what's bugging her and feel the expression of her displeasure. as well as reinforcing her position of authority over you and your closeness with a non-sexual but intimate activity."

Maintenance spanking is really discipline. as distinct from punishment. again according to blogger VeezKnight: "Discipline. by definition is on-going. and is routine-oriented in that it is recurs regularly. It is used to establish and maintain awareness of a specific set of rules. Punishment on the other hand involves action taken as retribution for infractions against established rules. It is dealt out as a consequence for specific. unacceptable behavior. As such. it should generally be more severe than discipline."

Punishment as Flip Side of Nurturing

Throughout these "P" Word blogposts. I have relied on other voices. because. I reiterate. none of this is a part of my own marriage. My wife leads be example. by hint. by directive when necessary. but never by coercion.

But I don't knock it for others. and. indeed. aspects of it I find daydream-worthy. And I can certainly agree with the on-topic insights of LFA advocate and psychologist Elise Sutton:

"Men need both the punisher and the nurturer. Most little boys were punished by their mothers but then also held and loved by the same woman who just disciplined them. Most men still long for that feeling. Love and punishment go hand and hand, as nurturing and discipline are the flip sides of the same coin of love. A man longs for both from the loving female... After he has suffered for you, he longs to be loved and nurtured by you. This process brings him inner peace and tranquility. He is a very lucky man because lots of men are seeking this from the woman they love but few get to experience it."

Before offering this analysis, Mme. Sutton cites an example of the husband-nurturing aspect of punishment from one of her female correspondents:

"One thing I have noticed is that [my husband] apologizes after the punishment and he usually wants to nurse on my breasts. After he undresses me I unhook the cups and allow him to suck while I hold him. He really seems to appreciate this. Since I have taken discipline to a new level, his behavior is even better... I find that if I am harsh when warranted, it has a lasting effect on him. He seems to be much more attentive to my needs and feelings."

There seems to be an overwhelming consensus among punitive practitioners that, properly and lovingly applied, these domestic rituals indeed bring couples closer—e.g., "[Punishment] taught me that she cares." It helps wives stop storing up resentments. The husband's shortcomings are addressed as they occur, the air is cleared, and the husband feels himself being placed back on the right track.

"I see spanking as an act of loving correction," a wife says in this spirit, "an action agreed by both parties as necessary for both parties to move on from something that was wrong."

Left to his own devices, he knows he is prone to succumb to a whole array of temptations that will could displease his wife and weaken his marriage, or at least undermine the loving female authority aspect of the marriage. In the words of the Lord's prayer. he is being led away from temptation and delivered from evil. or the temptation thereto.

But again. from the outside looking in. let me call on a regularly punished husband (cybernamed "Brad") for a penultimate word on this topic:

"In my opinion. corporal punishment serves three purposes. First. it hurts and that is a form of punishment. Second it 'cleanses' away the deed that he did to deserve the punishment. Third. the pain that he carries with him serves as a reminder to him of what is expected and what you can and will do to him. That's it. plain and simple. My wife and I don't consider correction cruel. She will tell me that she is sorry that she has to do this to me. But I want to live in a female-led relationship. and we both know that a 'You did not do this chore well' does not work."

The final word comes from another recipient of frequent wifely corrections: "Do I fear my wife?" he asks. "What sentient male does not?"

Comments:

Rex: I'm jealous of the spanked hubbies. Who among us doesn't crave such demonstrative feedback from our wives?

Mark: Me. too! No doubt you discerned the poorly concealed tone of envy in the post.

Ingrid Bellemare: I find that demerit marks. whereby my slave collects black marks for inappropriate behaviour. work very well. Punishment is administered according to the number of demerit marks.

Anonymous: I used to spank my husband by tying him face down on the bed with his hands tied to the headboard above him... I now realize that this is a men's fantasy. Now for punishment he gets denied orgasms for up to 2 months. and must spend a lot of his free time doing housework... No sport games on weekends if he has a punishment session coming to him. he does extended housework instead. His behavior has improved in a big way.

Wife In Control: Punishing your husband is easy. Restrict his orgasms to as few as possible. as stated here 10 a year is more than enough for any man... Make him do all of the housework. Very satisfying to watch your husband clean while you relax. read or watch tv... Tease him often and tell him there is no chance he will be cumming soon. that drives him crazy... Use your imagination. and if he suggests it as a punishment. don't do it because to him it probably won't be.

WORSHIPPING YOUR WIFE 2

Irene: I am a 20+ female from Asia. Presently I am into a very happy relationship with my boyfriend. I am learning a lot from all my other girlfriends from schools and now your site. I think it common to see boys serving their girlfriends in public these days... Before we became couples with my present Bf, I made him do almost every bit for me, if not, I would punish him. I even treat him quite badly at times but he still serve me and do to my demands. That's when my authority and dominant grows. Which I am also enjoying.

Do you see a difference society in the near future where woman rules and are in total control of the relationship? On the other hand, I am worried about seeing my 2 younger brothers as the slaves to their girlfriends.

Anonymous: Irene, it is great to see such a young woman exercising her dominant trait. You are doing your boyfriend a favor by making him serve you. Even if you don't stay with him, you have made him submissive for the next woman he will meet. Once a man becomes submissive, my husband says that they seldom have the desire to be dominant ever again. And that is so true with my husband. It took us many years (about 25) to find out our roles with each other, so you are off to a great start!

When I was in my 20's the male was always in charge, and I never thought that someday I would be punishing my husband because I am in charge and he now must please me. As for your brothers, communicate with their girlfriends or wives someday and try to drop hints to see if they have made your brothers submissive. You know your boyfriend is happy, otherwise he would have broken up with you. Your brothers will experience the same happiness.

My husband does wear a chastity device since I do not allow him to cum very often. Of course he begs, but I never give in. Try this on your boyfriend. You didn't state how you punish him, but I hope it's not by spanking. I learned with my husband that he liked that to much. Now I punish him my favorite way. He must strip naked and I bring him to a corner to stand in. I place a pair of my worn panties between his nose and the wall, tie his hands behind his back with about 16 inches of cord or scarf between his hands and command him to stay there—for 2 hours.

I can go out shopping, take a nap, or sun outside with no worry about him. If he moves away from the wall, the panties will drop to the floor and it will be impossible for him to pick them up and return to that position. (In case of an emergency, he can sit down, bring his tied hands down under his feet and untie himself. But this would have to be a real emergency. If the panties are on the ground when I return after 2 hours, he gets 2 more days at 2 hours each.)

Anonymous: After my husband read my comment post to Irene, he said it sounded like I have no sex life at all because I make him wait very long to cum. I do have a great sex life, although I am 55 years young. About once a week my husband provides me with a wonderful full body massage, uses

260

some of the many vibrator toys we own on me. and of course gives me intense oral sex.

Irene: Dear Anonymous Sister. I am still learning and I will put what I have learn to good use bit by bit and I will also share it with my school mates and friends. Sometime found myself being too cruel to him. it hurts me but I think I am also enjoy seeing him begging and suffering. Have I gone nuts?

Anonymous: Irene. No you haven't gone nuts. You are very young and just exploring domination with your boyfriend. You don't say how you administer punishment. but if your boyfriend is truly into female worship. there shouldn't be much punishment at all. We don't want slaves. we want a man who has decided that he wants to worship the woman he loves. I want my husband to wine and dine me. to do housework when he sees it's time to do it (ok. I do have to give a little reminder once every so often). and to pamper me with massages. the list goes on.

What I don't want is to stand over my husband with a whip in my hand making sure he washes the floors well. That's work for me and fantasy for him and most men I'm sure. So read this site well. and most of all have your boyfriend read every word of it as my husband does. Good luck. and keep exploring. you will find your own correct technique.

Another Anonymous: My wife and I have read all of the comments posted about punishing your husband. I believe that she thought she was the only one who actually punished her husband. she just couldn't get an idea if her friends did also. Well. now those comments opened her eyes. there are many wives punishing their man. and not only by withholding sex. That topic really sparked a good response.

16

CONCEAL OR REVEAL?

Going Public With Wife-Worship (4.15.08)

One of the obvious points of getting married is formalizing the relationship commitment in front of family, friends and surrounding society, including its institutions. A commitment that enfolds and protects the nascent family, which is the basic unit of a culture, a civilization.

Which, of course, is because the family protects and nurtures children, and launches them into responsible adulthood. As author George Gilder put it in his book, *Men and Marriage* (quoted on p. 6 of my book): "Women manipulate male sexual desire in order to teach men the long-term cycles of female sexuality and biology on which civilization is based."

In some primitive tribes, the man is required to pick up the child he has sired and acknowledge paternity and his commitment to support the child. Without that tightly woven social bond, connecting ejaculation with fatherhood, virile young males remain rogues, functioning as tribal gangs outside the social compact.

For men and women in wife-worship or wife-led marriages, "going public" can be extremely difficult and socially risky. Most often there is no surrounding social structure of friends, family and sympathetic institutions to sanction a role-reversal union. a lack that is sorely lamented by many FLR couples.

As Au876 wrote on Lady Misato's original Wife Worship forum several years back. "Deep down (and maybe not so deep) I think all of us want others to know about our devotion to our wives. That is why we like this forum. we are free to tell someone else. It excites us to have others know. Maybe someday it will become a more accepted lifestyle." Indeed. most of us are proud of serving our wonderful wives and wish we could tell the world of the joy and fulfillment this lifestyle brings us.

To take baby steps in that direction. more and more FLR couples seem to be renewing their marriage vows. this time with the wife pledging to "love. cherish and guide" and the husband to "love. honor. worship and obey." or variations thereof. While these marriage renewals are often intimate. private ceremonies. many of the participants would welcome an opportunity to make their affirmations as public declarations. with pride and joy and appropriate fanfare.

And some are doing exactly that.

Comments:

Stevielt: My wife and I have recently started to explore this new lifestyle of female-led marriage. We are making plans to move so we can live the life openly without scaring those that know us very well. This week she has taken a trip to investigate future living arrangements. When she gets back she said she would tell her best friend from work. I can't wait to see her friend after she knows my wife has full control over all aspects of my life. This is a very powerful feeling that I never thought of when we started this lifestyle.

Mark: Stevielt. there are many of us in wife-led marriages who secretly yearn to acknowledge our wife's leadership in the marriage. really sealing the deal. It is definitely one of those point-of-no return steps. I also envy you this further step that your wife contemplates. moving to a location where you can live your lifestyle openly and fully. Congratulations!

Stevielt: Well today is the day! My wife is having lunch with her best friend from work telling her about our new wife-led marriage. We had a wonderful session last night where she told me what she was going to tell her friend and what she thought her friend would say. I can't wait till tonight to hear about the actual conversation and what her friend's response was. My wife has control over all aspects of my life. her friend is going to be so jealous of her. I bet she tries to do the same with her boyfriend.

Mark: stevielt. I can't wait to hear the sequel.

Role-Reversal Rehearsal (6.13.08)

If you're addicted to those old '30s and '40s Broadway movies on AMC and TCM, you know that Broadway-bound shows always used to open "out of town," in order to work out the kinks.

FLR couples sometimes head out of town to work *in* the kinks. To try things, whether in private and public, that they might be afraid to try back home, where everybody knows them.

Except that, for FLR couples, "What happens in Vegas" doesn't necessarily stay in Vegas. A certain provocative practice might prove so much fun that she and he decide to bring it back home and incorporate it into the daily domesticity.

I was reminded of this not long ago in reading through posts from the old "Venus On Top Yahoo Discussion Group" (which recently evolved into a full-fledged FLR discussion board, "She Makes the Rules").

A guy asks: "Does anyone know of a place that supports FLR where the husband is allowed to serve his Wife while in the complex? Like a hotel or vacation spot?"

Another guy answers: "These places are everywhere. In every city and vacation spot you can think of. When you arrive at your destination, rush to open her car door for her. From this point on, pretend that you have class and that you would like your wife to have an unforgettable vacation. When you are with her in a public place, act in a way that will make her proud to be with you. Offer to do the things that she wants to do while on vacation and don't whine about it. Open doors for her, pull out her chair at supper... My point is that if you desire to give your wife a beautiful relaxing vacation, book it and prepare to treat her nice."

Then this followup comment: "When my wife and i go on trips we both check in and she will send me to get the bags and unpack while she checks out the hotel. When she gets back to the room everything is in place."

Which reminded me of a like-minded post by Au876 from Lady Misato's original Wife Worship board:

"We went to visit some of my wife's girlfriends at a lake cabin a couple of years ago. We had to take our own sheets and etc. One of the first things I did after getting the car unloaded was to make up our bed and put her clothes away. Later we were all sitting around talking. My wife asked me 'Have you made up my bed yet?' One of the ladies started to laugh like that was a stupid thing to expect of a man. But I quickly responded telling her yes and I had hung up all of clothes too...

"My wife was real proud of me. The lady that laughed made some sort of comment about what a good husband I was. and my wife responded saying something like. 'He knows what is expected of him.'

"I was not embarrassed. I was proud of myself. I had done what I was supposed to do. The fact my wife asked me was a sure sign she did not intend to keep my status a secret from them. The fact I had already done it was a sure sign to her I was not ashamed of my status."

Another member of Misato's original husbands' forum. who posted under the name of "Johann." described an out-of-town tryout where his wife and he flirted with mild public humiliation:

"I kept silent and followed closely to her left rear. I stepped ahead to open doors. I never realized that waitresses tend to ignore other women. But I would not respond even by eye contact. My mentrice ordered everything and soon the waitresses got the drift. I think they'd seen it before. The waitress would ask: 'Are you ready to order. sir?' My wife would answer. 'Yes. he will have the Crab Louis and a glass of Pinot Grigio. Failing that. a dry Riesling. followed by coffee. after dinner.' That was the general tone.

"It was good for me to enter the role publicly and privately. I spoke very few words all weekend. offered no suggestions and was treated like a pet and a servant. It was good for her and even more so for me. I recommend this. No, I do not think we im-posed on anyone. Some people were disoriented when they spoke to me. I would look at my Lady and she would answer."

"Female Led" is SOP, home and away, for fdhousehusband, who authored the now-discontinued blog, "Her Househusband's Life."

He regularly chronicled his daily life, including holidays and getaways, with candid replays of all his submissive routines. As he explained a couple years ago in a report on a family outing to Disney World: "Although i didn't have to do all the cooking, cleaning, and other housework like at home, i am still bound to follow Her Rules of Behaviour when we are on a trip."

Fd (just like Au876), upon arrival at a hotel or resort, would promptly unpack for everyone, while his wife—and kids, if they were along—headed off for the pool, the lake, the seashore or perhaps the nearest mall.

Happy traveling!

Wife-Led Shopping – The Ultimate Test, Part 1 (7.1.09)

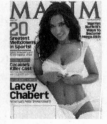

In an interview in *Maxim* magazine [January, 2007], actress Lacey Chabert was asked how a guy could impress her. She answered: "The true test is if he's willing to go shopping with me. Will you go shopping, and will you hold the purse while I'm looking around and trying stuff on? He should be interactive and make comments, too, rather than reiterating how bored he is."

Is Ms. Chabert right? Does co-ed shopping constitute a "true test" of romantic chivalry and "female-led"? What's so difficult about publicly escorting the object of one's affection into the retail depths of the Estrogen Zone (especially if one is being leashed and led by a delicious creature like Ms. Chabert)?

Yet, for a surprising number of guys, even would-be submissive guys, the female-led shopping experience can be alarming. It is almost as if they fear they will never emerge again, at least not with full macho functionality intact.

And maybe they're right to be wary, even fearful. Witness what happened to one poor doofus after who knows how many wife-led shopping expeditions: "I enjoy shopping with my wife now, watching 'chick' flicks, etc. Is this normal?"

So let's talk about it. After all, one of the chief purposes of this blog, like my book (inspired by Lady Misato's original online support group for husbands), is to encourage guys, married or single, to share their woman-worshipping dreams and yearnings, along with any associated fears.

That was the spirit in which, around a decade ago, I posted the following confession on Lady M's Husbands' Forum:

"One area in which I've been a typical inconsiderate husband is shopping. Always looking for a place to sit down, wondering how long we're going to be in a particular store, looking bored, massively fatigued. Like many husbands, I even have to be dragged into men's departments to replace my own wardrobe, kept in the changing booth while my wife hands me stuff, over my protests that I don't need anything! It got to where she would ask me if I wouldn't mind if she looked around a bit before we left the mall, or would it be okay if we went into a particular store, or up to the next level. What an inconsiderate boob I've been.

"I've decided to reform. Okay, it's not ever going to be my favorite thing. But pleasing her is. And I'm going to make it clear that from now on, I'll be happy to accompany her into any store, she can shop as long as she wants, I won't complain, look bored, etc. I'll be right with her, offering an opinion if asked, delighted to be beside her, carrying parcels, etc. About time, too."

Have I kept that resolve? I wish I could say yes. Truth is, I'm still a mall-walking foot-dragger, looking for a place to plop down, preferably in front of a TV showing a game, any game.

Not so for another member of Lady Misato's forum, the oft-quoted Au876, who was quick to offer support for my resolve to reform by sharing his own story:

"I had the same shopping problems in the past. Mostly shopping is just not a 'man' thing. We know what we want, go get it and get out. But that has changed now. I go with my wife (if invited -- sometimes she likes to go alone). I carry the packages. The last time she went clothes shopping - about two months ago - she got a bunch of clothes to try on. They only allowed two things in the dressing room at a time. I stood outside her dressing cubicle. She'd try on something, send me to get a different size or color, put it in the 'to buy' stack or back on the rack. Several times she sent me to get a certain color shoe to see how the dress went with them. Several other customers were struggling with trying on clothes without the help of their husbands. I found myself busting with pride to be so much help to my wife."

Au876's description of catering to his wife while shopping came as a revelation to me at the time. What a pioneer! I thought. What I was promising to do, this man had actually done, in defiance of masculine nature. If he could do this impossible thing, then other guys could, too.

And, indeed, I began to come across quotes from other husbands who, like wild broncos broken to the saddle, had learned to follow their wives obediently not only into department stores, but into all the feminine departments thereof, to fetch and carry and never speak a discouraging word. I saved a lot of these posts, and I offer them here as evidence of what a man can achieve if his wife sets his mind to it:

Let's start with several examples from the old Spousechat board:

Charles: "Once Lisa was trying on some skirts at a department store. The saleswoman was assisting her and I was sitting in the 'husbands' chair with Lisa's packages, purse, etc. The saleswoman said that perhaps she should try a size 4. Lisa, without even looking in my direction, points in my direction and snaps her fingers. I immediately go to her and she simply says

CONCEAL OR REVEAL?

'go find this in a size 4'. The saleswoman smiled and I heard her say. 'Boy. he sure is handy.'"

Ms. Lynda: *"The company I am working for sent me to a town about 180 miles away from where I live. We had lunch and did some shopping before we returned to the home office. Mr. Lynda followed us through the shopping mall and carried out packages. When I tried on a new outfit. I had him hold my purse."*

Charles: *"Ms. Lynda. I frequently accompany my wife shopping. and on occasion. one or two of her friends will shop with her and I will happily accompany them. In order to make their shopping more enjoyable. not only will I carry their packages, but I will even take the outfits Lisa wants to try on to the dressing room for her and stand in line to pay so she doesn't have to. I'll hold her purse and her friends' purses if they want me to. I've never received anything but compliments from women. customers and salespeople alike. On occasion. a man will say something like. 'Boy. does she have you trained.' usually jokingly. Any man who is saying this to me is probably out shopping with his wife as well and is probably also doing as he is told.*

"When shopping with Lisa. I cater to her every demand without the slightest complaint. I even get on my knees and take off and put on her shoes for her when she is shoe shopping. Once. a saleswoman was joking with Lisa as I was trying a pair of shoes on her. The saleswoman asked if Lisa makes me kiss her feet. so I playfully kissed Lisa's instep. both of them were entertained by this."

Another aspect of wife-led shopping. of course. is for the modern knight errant to be sent forth by his damsel in quest of needed feminine items:

Mr. Lynda: *"As I begin to do more and more of the shopping by myself. I am having a little problem buying tampons and other feminine products. So far. Lynda has always been with me. How do you cope with everyone looking at you?"*

Charles: *"I have no problem buying most of Lisa's personal products. even pantyhose or hair and skin care products at the*

269

salon, but I must confess that the feminine hygiene products I do still find incredibly embarrassing to buy. The way to do it is to just mix them in with a large food order at the grocery store, and stay away from the younger checkout employees. The older ones will never say anything, the younger ones have."

Charles, who, at the urging of Ms. Lynda began calling himself "Mr. Lisa," goes on to describe one of these solo shopping expeditions in quest of personal items:

"This morning Lisa gave me a shopping list which required a trip to Victoria's Secret to get her four pair of pantyhose (Lisa really likes their pantyhose, although at $14 a pair, I think they are expensive). I approached the counter and told the saleswoman why I was there, and of course, she smiled and thought it was great. Two customers at the counter also thought it was fantastic that my wife sent me out to buy her pantyhose... Then it was off to the hair salon to get Lisa's shampoo and styling gel..."

Another Spousechatter, styling himself "Uxorious Husband," takes up this same theme: "Learn to shop for her; learn what she likes, what colors, styles. Yes, you do have to be trained! That means going to shop with her over and over again, no more helpless mall bench sitting. No, sir. Go to every shop, ask detailed questions. Let her try on the whole store if she likes. Smell, look, taste, compare. Your style should be an extension of her style."

Au876 also recommends taking careful notes on a wife's sizes and preferences as an excellent way for a husband to make the most of mall outings (and earn future bonus points):

"I watched her like a hawk when she took me shopping. She would pick up things and make comments. To me this was a window into her likes and dislikes. I checked out her closet, not just for the obvious things like shoe size, but what colors were in her palate and what stores she shopped at."

Fdhousehusband (whose discontinued blog, "Her househusband's life," is sorely missed) makes the same point: "I am amazed how many males do not know their wives' dress size, her shoe size, her color preferences, her food preferences, etc... I want to find out everything i can about Her. The more I know, the better I can serve her."

Offering one's opinions is fine, to a point. Charles, if you recall, had reservations about the practicality of some of Lisa's preferences (VS Pantyhose @ $14 a pair). One wonders if he ever actually expressed these opinions to Lisa, as fdhousehusband dared to do to his wife-leader, with immediate consequences:

"Like most of America, we spent the day after Thanksgiving shopping. I followed along mostly to carry the bags. I made the mistake of saying that I thought the some of the items were too expensive. She didn't change her demeanor but continued to smile and enjoy the shopping experience with our daughters. When the girls were both in the changing room, she took me aside out of hearing range from anyone and chastised me. 'Listen, I make almost all the money for this family. It is my money to spend as I see fit. Understand?' she said. I apologized and she turned to walk back to the changing room. I meekly followed her carrying her bags of purchases."

I wrote that Au876's description of catering to his wife while shopping came as a revelation to me. Later I learned that Elise Sutton, that intrepid Internet pioneer of Loving Female Authority, had earlier formulated female-led shopping as one of the procedures she offered to wives just exploring the lifestyle: "Elise Sutton's Procedure No. 10: Public Outing (a trip to a shopping mall was never more fun)"

One husband described Ms. Sutton's outing thus: "A woman's day shopping trip, with the woman dressed seductively, or in leather skirt or boots, anything powerful. The male follows behind carrying packages and taking orders. The woman drops hints to cashiers, interested shoppers or women waiting in line. If any are interested, again they are explained the dynamics of the relationship."

Judging from Elise Sutton's "Real Stories" archives, there has been no shortage of wives eager to give Procedure No. 10 a trial run, with results gratifying to both parties. An example:

"Dear Elise, I followed your exercise and I made my husband walk behind me and carry my purchases. I was nervous at first, but as the day went on I grew very comfortable and confident. I bought a lot of clothes and other things. I was really having a great time shopping, as this was the first time I can ever remember that my husband wasn't bitching and complaining the whole time. He couldn't because he wasn't allowed to speak."

More recently Ms. Sutton has suggested a refinement to female-led shopping, especially when mall parking is at a premium. The wife can "send her husband early in the morning, before the mall opens and have him get a spot near the door. Then when his [wife] shows up, communicating via a cell phone so she can find him, she can take the place he has reserved for her... Better yet, have him go and park far away after she has taken his spot and he can join her in the mall and carry her purchases."

And perhaps carry more than just her purchases, as this observer notes: "Have you ever gone to the mall to people watch? How many times have you noticed a male following a female as she is leading the way? Sometimes he will even hold her purse for her!"

In fact, carrying milady's handbag seems to be part and parcel of the whole FLR shopping experience, according to much of the online testimony I've collected from proud husbands and demanding wives:

"My wife hands her purse to me frequently when errands/shopping - nobody takes notice. She likes being out and about and so this is going to happen frequently as a matter of course. A few times she called out to me in apparel stores to hold her things so she could try some stuff on. Then she would pile stuff in my arms as she went through her various outfits."

"Last Sunday, at a large outlet shopping center north of New York City, I watched two men laden with shopping bags and their girlfriend's purses as they walked from store to store. The women carried absolutely nothing. The men seemed quite content with their beasts-of-burden status and the women were free to talk and walk without distraction."

"My wife took me shopping with her on Saturday. For an entire day. I follow her around. holding the clothes that she selects from the racks. I hold her purse (and sometimes her shoes) while she goes into the dressing room. I carry her selections to the register and pay for them. Then. of course. I carry all her bags. I take her to lunch. I'm basically her fawning. pussy-whipped husband for the entire shopping day. "

"We went shopping two nights ago at a local mall. I saw a lot of men sitting on benches in the pedestrian areas waiting for their wife. Not me. I was following in her footsteps carrying all the packages and most of the time her purse. My shoulders and back ached by the time we got home. Then I had to rub and feet and give her a massage. I really feel good about myself right now. I feel so useful to her."

"On Monday. we were shopping and I held her coat on my arm and wore her purse over my shoulder the whole time we were in the mall. Very often she will just hand me her purse to hold."

Starting to get the picture? Just to make sure. in the continuation of this two-part post. I'm going to offer additional examples of husbands happily harnessed to their shopaholic wives.

Comments:
Whatevershesays: I think all men in wife led marriages should carry the bags. open the doors. etc. I do it for my wife but she doesn't want me to carry her purse. she thinks it's silly and too over the top.

My favorite moments are when she walks up to a door and then just stands there and waits for me to walk around her and open it. Very obvious. Another is when I walk ahead of her then she stops and looks at me. I then have to go back and stand behind her. Oh and how could I forget the "He will pay for it"? And the "Pay for it. I'll be at (the next store)"? But my all time favorite is while we were at the cashier. my wife noticed it was a hand-wash only item. And right in front of the cashier she told me that I was to hand-wash it and it was my responsibility.

Mark: I don't often get the privilege of being taken shopping by my wife these days. More often she will take one or the other of the kids. or go shopping alone. So I have to defer to all you husbands who are being mall-trained by their wives.

Wife-Led Shopping – The Ultimate Test, Part 2 (7.7.09)

In Chapter 5 ("Pampering and Pitching In") of my book, I quote an ecstatic wife describing a few of the many benefits of wife worship: "Gone are the days when my husband just plops in front of the TV after work. Now he actually looks for opportunities to do household chores, volunteers to go shopping with me and helps me with carrying the purchases…"

But these husbands do more than accompany their wives to the nearest fashion marketplace and dutifully carry her accumulating parcels. Here is a sampling of devoted hubbies ready, willing or simply required to go the extra mall-mile:

"Take her shopping whenever and wherever she wants to go, carrying her bags for her, open doors for her, and pay the bills!"

"He should be taken shopping with you and allowed to hold your purse while you try on any number of items or test cosmetics for a perfect color or gloss. I have done both any number of times and it really demonstrates to her and everyone else for that matter your complete devotion to her. I have stood in front of a cosmetic counter for at least 30 minutes, holding her purse the whole while."

"When I'm with her, she relegates me to the dutiful husband, who is expected to carry her bags and quite frankly, just do as I'm told. If she's trying something on in a change room, she'll have me holding her purse, her bags, and I'm not to move from the spot she puts me in. Often she wants me at arms length, in case she needs my opinion, or perhaps to fetch another size. The saleswomen probably figures I'm just henpecked, but the reality is this is all an expression of my utter devotion to my wife."

In fact, shopping with the wife seems to be a standard component of "dutiful" hubby-ness. To rank husbands on a devoted-

and-dutiful scale of 1 through 10. one survey asked: "Would you go shopping with your wife whenever she wished. since she enjoyed it. and stand around while she looked at clothes or shoes for whatever. to please her. despite the fact that you find it boring and would rather do something else?"

Most wife-led husbands writing about this topic have learned to love these outings. Like these guys:

"I always feel ecstatic when my wife invites me to go shopping with her. Especially when she tries on new clothes. It gives me a chance to be the 'mirror on the wall' and tell her she is the best-looking woman in the mall in that new outfit. This is not untruthful because she never picks out ugly clothes and she is a very good looking woman. I'm never be too tired to appreciate her beauty in a new outfit and to tell here so. no matter how late in the evening it might be. I also carry the packages for her. of course."

"She was shopping for clothes one afternoon while on the trip. Of course I was right there helping holding packages and helping her. She had picked out several blouses to try on. The sales clerk warned her they had to be hand-washed. My wife laughed and said. 'I don't worry about washing instructions. that is my husband's job.' The clerk said she wished she had a husband like that. They stood there and talked a few minutes with my wife telling a complete stranger in my presence how I did all the cooking. cleaning. laundry and etc. I have to admit I was proud of myself."

"Next to me another guy was commenting to me about both of us had some nice-looking ladies to attend to and noted that we both were blessed with ladies who liked to show off when shopping."

But occasionally you come across a reluctant escort who boasts about going along against all his macho inclinations. and maybe thinks he should get combat pay for his efforts: "Over the next few weeks. I found myself being attentive to my wife almost every night. I even went mall shopping with her on a regular basis: something I really hate."

Some women are tolerant of guys who walk into stores and park themselves on the first available chair: "My husband especially loves shoe shopping because he knows there will always be a place for him to sit. Why don't more women's fashion stores have boyfriend chairs for the guys?"

For many other women, however, hanging back, looking bored, toe-tapping, watch-checking, heaving weary sighs, all constitute unacceptable behavior, not only in shopping but in any wife-led activity. The ideal would seem to be enthusiastic and helpful participation by hubby in all facets of the shopping experience.

The following quotes illustrate how acceptable or admirable male participation is encouraged by some wives (and how anything less is discouraged and even penalized):

"Jane called out to me, 'We have forgotten this and that, do you want to go back to the shop?' When I replied, 'Not really' in a less than enthusiastic voice, Jane was quick to add, 'But you're going, aren't you.' Realising my mistake, I said, 'Yes, of course,' and so it was that I had to go back, because Jane had insisted. (From the blog, "At All Times")

"If we are out alone shopping and I am less than attentive, she has been known to send me to the car to wait for her and it has been hours that I've waited."

"The past weekend we were in my wife's hometown. We were out shopping. She kept running into old acquaintances. I was not part of the conversations, not even introduced. I simply stood back, held the bags, and smiled."

"I follow her around shopping malls carrying her bags, and coffee and coat, while trying to keep up to her and open doors for her while she waits for me while tapping her toes."

"When we are together at the mall, I give her my undivided attention and I am usually always at her side and prepared to do her bidding. She prefers it this way."

"Once we were in a shoe store for quite some time, and she finally picked out what she wanted and as we approached the register she said, 'Pay for these, I'll be in the next store.' One of my favorites was when we were shopping for a blouse. She was about 20 feet away and I held one up and said, 'How about this one?' She responded, 'No, it's just like the one I own, and if you'd keep up with ironing, we wouldn't need it.' There must have been about 5 women who heard that!" (From the "Whatevershesays" blog.)

"In one store I was handed a pair of stockings and several new pairs of panties that Jane wanted to buy. I had to carry these around the shop for sometime as Jane browsed for other items. In one part of the shop, there were three young, smartly dressed and particularly attractive girls all out shopping together. I think that they noticed me following Jane around, carrying her new underwear. Although they didn't say anything I could see that they thought this was highly amusing." (From the "At All Times" blog.)

"My wife went to the underwear dept. and picked out three pair. A clerk was there helping her and said she didn't know if it made any difference or not but those needed to be hand-washed. My wife handed them to me and said 'All mine have to be hand-washed.' There was no doubt what she meant."

"My wife yelled out for me to get a different size while she was in a dressing room. When handed a shoe by a saleslady and asked if she liked it, my wife responded by silently handing me the shoe to put on her foot. I was carrying 6 shopping bags while she was empty handed. And I was then told to find her size in a particular outfit in a matching color."

"Today, once my nail polish is dry and the kitchen is clean, my husband will bathe me in a milk bath and then he will accompany me and a friend of mine shopping at the mall. Not only will he follow behind us carrying our bags, but his allowance will buy our lunch, though he doesn't know that yet."

"In a store once, I saw a young college-age woman and her boyfriend shopping for shoes. This young woman was having a conversation on her cell phone and she was discussing, not that I was eavesdropping, some kind of a complicated engineering research project, sounded like something to do with biomedical engineering. As she was heavily involved in her conversation, she'd point to various shoes she wanted to try on and her boy-friend would get them for her in her size, and try them on her feet." [From the Spousechat archives]

"When we are in public together, such as on a shopping trip, her authority is obvious. I hold the door open for her getting in and out of the car. If we are in a store I follow behind her and push the shopping cart and I carry the packages. She carries the money and always handles the purchase transaction. I dress and groom well for these occasions and am always polite and friendly. This kind of behavior can sometimes have the effect of making other women jealous of my wife. Of course, she loves it when that happens, and I am likely to be rewarded later."

For one extremely dutiful househusband, just being taken out a shopping expedition with his wife-leader qualifies as a special treat:

"My husband has been a home-bound house-husband for more than a year now, doing the housework, the yard and pool work, while I work 40 hours a week, bringing home the bacon. He gets to go with me to town for shopping on weekends, and sometimes on a weeknight after I get home from work. But the rest of the time he's my sweet little 'Peter, Peter, Pumpkin-eater.' I keep him in our 'pumpkin shell' and there he stays, very well."

I'll close with another quote from Au876 (again posting on Lady Misato's original Yahoo! husbands' forum). He describes what just might be the ultimate wife-directed shopping trip:

"Friday night my wife was reading the paper. A local depart-ment store was having a big sale on women's clothing (what else is new?). Anyway, she saw several dresses advertised that she liked. She already had plans for Saturday and didn't want to change them. So she said she wanted me to go to the sale, buy each one of the dresses in several different sizes and bring them home for her to try on. I could take back the ones that she didn't like. She also suggested I pick out some scarves and maybe a purse or two that I thought would go with them.

"So I spent most of Saturday afternoon shopping for her

clothes. I got the clerk to help me pick out some extra things to go with the dresses. She tried them on Sunday and is keeping two dresses plus several of the other items. I am taking the un-wanted items back this afternoon. My wife said this was a great way to shop and she didn't know why she hadn't thought of it sooner.

"I had to agree. She loves to shop but she often does not have the time. She was able to take advantage of the sale and still do what she had planned Saturday. I felt like I had been a real help to her and it was a step forward for me in our relationship."

Comments:
Worship Her: As a bonus. my wife now takes me into the dressing room as she tries on new clothes so she doesn't have to walk out of it to show me and get my opinion. So I get to see her strip down to her bra and panties sev-eral times and get to ogle her fabulous body.

LadyDiandl: I love it when Lady Di lets me accompany her shopping. It is a delightful feeling to hold her purse while she's in the fitting room. We've also done shoe shopping as well. The feeling of kneeling in front of her and dressing her feet to try on shoes is indescribable. It's even sweeter when other shoppers notice.

Remedial Chivalry (7.16.08)

Even now. with my golden years in sight. I still yearn to achieve some goals left over from boyhood and teenage years. Oh. I've given up on running a 5-minute mile or bench pressing 300 pounds. But I still have designs on someday cruising the Danube from Vienna to Varna on the Black Sea. and maybe learning enough Homeric Greek to work my way through the *Odyssey* in the original.

Near the top of this long-running resolve list is an item I should have accomplished decades ago. back when I pledged my heart to the girl who would rule my heart for the rest of my life:

Resolved: to be a better and more attentive escort to my wife.

Embarrassing Confession: Despite this sincere resolve, I too often neglect my wife at cocktail parties, wedding receptions, and similar social functions. There I stand, doping off, unaware that her wineglass is empty or that the waiter just forgot to serve her dessert.

Or maybe I just forget to pull out her chair or remove her coat or wrap. And, yikes, did I just say the wrong thing to the wrong person, or forget a name and face I should darned well know? Yep, and now my wife is having to rescue me again from appearing like a social doofus.

This is unacceptable behavior for any husband, let alone one who professes to worship, adore and serve his better half. By now I should be like Au876, a paragon of chivalry according to his years-ago postings on Lady Misato's Wife Worship Forum:

"Showing Your Worship of Her in Public: I have been trying to make an example of our marriage in the presence of other couples by the way I treat my wife. Treat her like she is the most important and most special person in the world (after all, she is). Your wife will glow in that and appreciate the way you behave in front of her or your friends. There is a tendency among men to put down their wife in public. The exact opposite should be the case."

Obviously, I need help. So I've been collecting some do's and don'ts from Au and other attentive husbands, like this:

"You will want to find out how she will expect you to comport yourself in public. She will likely expect you to open doors for her, stand when she enters a room, light her cigarette, and perform other acts of chivalry. She may have different protocols for you depending on where you are and with whom.

"When we are together I give her my undivided attention and I am usually always at her side and prepared to do her bidding. She prefers I stay silent unless spoken to."

Is that excessive deference on the part of a husband? Well, how I wish I'd observed those strictures at a recent function. I actually interrupted my wife when she was talking to a woman across our table. She turned at looked at me in incredulity and annoyance. then snapped. "I'm talking. don't interrupt." I stammered back: "I just wanted to ask if you wanted another glass of wine."

See. even when I'm trying to be chivalrous. I klutz it up!

But some guys get it. like the husband who called himself "Mr. Lisa" on the old Spouseclub message board (several years defunct):

"My job at the party will to remain at [my mother-in-law's] side as her personal waiter for the afternoon/evening. Lisa thinks this will be a good experience for me. and that it should not be humiliating to me to have to serve in this manner. and I guess it isn't really."

But no spouse. I think. gets it better than Fdhousehusband. who describes the instructions he was given by his executive wife when he escorted her to a corporate event:

"'I hate carrying a purse to these functions [his wife told him]. Put these in your pockets.' i dutifully found a place in my pockets for Her cell and all Her other odds and ends. 'you will be my walking purse tonight. I want you close by in case I need anything. understand? Stay at my side. smile and look charming... your job tonight is to convince them that you are the perfect supporting spouse whose job it is to take care of My house and My kids so that I can focus on my job 100%.'"

Which is just what he did: "[As] She worked the room. i stayed at Her right elbow. slightly behind Her. just where Her purse would be. my pockets were bulging with Her stuff and i found myself getting hard at the thought of being nothing more than Her purse tonight. i fetched Her drinks and hors d'oeuvres and remained at Her beck and call all night."

If you consult the transcripts from the old Spousechat message board (reprinted on my blogsite). you can read the voluminous postings of Ms. Lynda. a dynamic young woman who launched herself into an upwardly mobile executive job right out of college. taking her boyfriend along for the ride. marrying him and turning him into a full-time "subordinate and submissive" househusband, whom she referred to as "Mr. Lynda":

"Just as some men enjoy the public adoration of their wives, I think I will enjoy the very public adoration of Mr. Lynda when it becomes even more popular to do so… As people become more comfortable with our life, it would be nice to have Mr. Lynda admit in public that it is my earnings that supply our lifestyle, that I am the boss at home, and that he enjoys being a corporate spouse."

On a popular Yahoo! FLR blog (authored by "happydomwife" Barbara), I found among the "10 golden rules" of proper gentlemanly behaviour one that I should absolutely commit to memory:

"You make sure that no woman remains with an empty glass! It is your duty to always keep an eye on it and ask a lady politely if she would like a refill or something else."

Followed by:

"You do not eat in presence of women unless every woman has been served some food and is eating."

There are many more chivalric rules in the same vein, followed by this summation:

"Gentlemanly behaviour in a man for me has to express and radiate his genuine respect for womanhood. Just think of the good old days when a proper gentleman was throwing himself in the dirt so a lady could walk over him without getting her feet and shoes dirty!

"I told my darling that in his presence a woman should never have to do menial tasks such as carrying stuff (other than her handbag), cleaning up dirt, fetch things etc.! All those things are his duty! Furthermore I expect him to do those duties with eagerness, thus expressing that he considers it a privilege just to be allowed to be in our presence!"

Amen! I mean, Ah, Women!

Comments:
Enoch: This is an area I am actually pretty good at. Since I'm not that comfortable at big parties or events, I tend to stay close to my wife and to

make sure she is taken care of. I'm much happier standing with her and talking to another couple or individual than I am talking to someone on my own.

I feel the same way [fd does] when my wife hands me her purse when we are at the mall. And I have to say I really enjoy carrying her bags for her. I guess since I get a kick out of it. I am attentive to make sure I always do. or at least always offer.

Whatevershesays: I just try and remember when we were first dating and that usually covers most issue such as door-holding. etc.

Mark: Why didn't I say that? Why haven't I behaved like that? It's exactly what I preach.

17

WOMAN WORSHIP IN THE MEDIA

RLS and the Enchanted Isle (1.5.07 – my first blog-post)

I begin with this delicious tribute to the woman-worshipping lifestyle from Robert Louis Stevenson, than whom no one crafted more elegant English:

"Harry was transferred to the feminine department, where his life was little short of heavenly. He was always dressed with uncommon nicety, wore delicate flowers in his button-hole, and could entertain a visitor with tact and pleasantry. He took a pride in servility to a beautiful woman; received Lady Vandeleur's commands as so many marks of favour; and was pleased to exhibit himself before other men in his character of male lady's-maid and man milliner. Nor could he think enough of his existence from a moral point of view. Wickedness seemed to him an essentially male attribute, and to pass one's days with a delicate woman, and principally occupied about trimmings, was to inhabit an enchanted isle among the storms of life."

(From *New Arabian Nights*, "Story of the Bandbox")

It is safe to say that the author shared some of Harry's female-celebrating tendencies. Anyone who doubts need only consult any RLS biography and turn to the chapters dealing with his courtship of, and by, Fannie Osborne.

Near the Center of the Feminine Mystery (1.7.07)

Shortly after posting the Stevenson quote ("The Enchanted Isle" below) I began to hear faint echoes in memory. A quick search of some old files turned up the following from an obviously enraptured husband to an old (and now defunct) Yahoo! group (entitled something like "Happy Wives and Trained Husbands"):

"[My wife] has arrived home and my heart is fluttering with excitement! I hurry to do her bidding. I do not feel complete until she is home. I'm near the center of the feminine mystery, an intimate part of the life of a beautiful woman. So close to her, caring only for her comfort and happiness."

I am reminded not only of Stevenson's "enchanted isle among the storms of life," but of how love transforms surroundings. I remember the special magic that pervaded the apartments and neighborhoods of certain females in my younger days, even the freeway offramps leading to these sacred precincts. It is the way Freddy Eynsford-Hill felt "on the street where you live," as a lovesick sentry posted outside Prof. Higgins' home, hoping for just a glimpse of Liza Dolittle.

Now, of course, her abode is mine and ours, and the covered playground of two kids. And yet everything about it reminds me that it is *she* who created it, who is its head and heart, the leader who holds us all in her loving embrace. I give thanks each day that I live here with her, and them, in her "enchanted isle," "near the center of the feminine mystery, an intimate part of the life of a beautiful woman."

A Bit of Dickens (4.5.07)

Dickens is known for angelic heroines, who, by age 17, are em-
bodiments of human perfection. There is no shortage, either, of
young men afflicted with unrequited adoration for these para-
gons—or for anti-paragons (see below). Dickens himself, as a
young man, mooned over and pursued a young lady in this fashion.

One such idealized young woman is the title character of *Little Dorrit*. But it is her older sister, the vain and lovely Miss
Fanny, who ensnares the luckless Sparkler:

"Mr. Sparkler entered on an evening of agony... But he had
two consolations at the close of the performance. [Miss Fanny]
gave him her fan to hold while she adjusted her cloak, and it was
his blessed privilege to give her his arm down-stairs again.
These crumbs of encouragement, Mr. Sparkler thought, would
just keep him going; and it is not impossible that [Miss Fanny]
thought so too... Mr. Sparkler put on another heavy set of fetters
over his former set, as he watched her radiant feet twinkling
down the stairs beside him."

In short order, Fanny's conquest of Sparkler is complete, and
he is reduced to groveling.

Of course, Miss Fanny is not an isolated case in Dickens'
novels. Pip, the beloved hero of *Great Expectations*, is "brought
up by hand" by his sister, Mrs. Joe Gargery, who was "much in
the habit of laying it upon her husband as well as upon me." Pip
and Joe both take to cowering in the chimney corner to stay out
of her reach—and the reach of "Tickler," "a wax-ended piece of
cane, worn smooth by collision with my tickled frame."

A final comment on the Victorian wife-led marriage I draw
from Chapter 6 of *Nicholas Nickleby*:

"It is not for me to say by what means, or by what degrees,
some wives manage to keep down some husbands as they do,
although I may have my private opinion on the subject, and may
think that no Member of Parliament ought to be married, inas-
much as three married members out of every four, must vote

according to their wives' consciences (if there be such things). and not according to their own. All I need say. just now. is. that the Baroness Von Koeldwethout somehow or other acquired great control over the Baron Von Koeldwethout. and that. little by little. and bit by bit. and day by day. and year by year. the baron got the worst of some disputed question. or was slyly unhorsed from some old hobby: and that by the time he was a fat hearty fellow of forty-eight or thereabouts. he had no feasting. no revelry. no hunting train. and no hunting—nothing in short that he liked. or used to have: and that. although he was as fierce as a lion. and as bold as brass. he was decidedly snubbed and put down. by his own lady. in his own castle of Grogzwig."

Cool-Whipped (2.4.07)

Is it cool to be "whipped." as in "pussywhipped"? That's certainly one of the minor messages imparted in the girls' gymnastics movie. *Stick It* (2006). My 12-year-old daughter liked the movie in the theater and now is renting the DVD.

A couple of young guys. one blonde. the other dark-haired. friends of the main-character gymnast. hang around the periphery of the story. cracking wise. but also cheering wholeheartedly during the girls' competitions. One of the boys is clearly smitten with another of the leotard-clad girls. a prototypical bitch (as played by Vanessa Lengies: the boy is played John Patrick Amedori. see photo).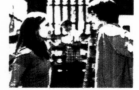

In fact. the blond boy calls her a bitch to her face. She asks the smitten friend. "Do *you* think I'm a bitch?" He answers. "No. I mean. yeah. but I don't have a problem with that. unlike some other guys." (Glancing at his buddy.)

The girl. evidently pleased with his response. proceeds to invite herself to his prom, tells him when and where to pick her up and not to forget to buy her a corsage, then turns on her heel, gymnastically, and prances away. Blonde guy tells his lovestruck friend, "Dude, you are so whipped!"

The friend answers, "What is wrong with that—ever?"

Blonde guy, apparently considering the ramifications of being "whipped" for the first time in his life, finally nods in agreement. Like, yeah, what *is* wrong with being whipped?

Just asking.

Josie and Clemmie (7.31.08)

I'm featuring passages from two writers, one famous, one obscure, both describing eerily similar scenes of a willful, authoritarian young woman laying down the law to her soon-to-be husband.

The first is from a short story called "Walter" by a gifted writer pseudonymed "Eosuchus." Google will direct you to his blog, where you can find a sampling of his short femdom fiction. I've trimmed the passage below slightly for space.

The second excerpt is from *Clemmie*, a 1958 paperback original by the late, great mystery-thriller novelist John D. MacDonald, author of the well-known Travis McGee series and a particular favorite of mine.

Wouldn't it be delicious to have Clemmie and Josie meet and compare dominant notes? Or, alternatively, the men under their thumbs, Walter and Fitz?

Josie (from "Walter" by Eosuchus):

Josie [Brooks] knew she had work yet to do, before [Walter] would be worth marrying. She had a very clear picture of the kind of marriage she wanted. She would be the Queen of that household. also the Judge and the CEO.

"You're going to be my lovely husband. Walter. You'll do what I want and you'll obey me in everything. I will take good care of you. my darling. but you will submit to me and serve me in all things... [You'll] change your name when we're married... Yes. your male pride is gonna take a beating." She giggled and pouted those big red lips at him. "That's not the only thing that's going to get a beating. either." she said slyly and moved across the room and sat beside him. crossing her legs and smoothing her skirt... "You come here now and get over my knee. You know what I have to do."

"Josie. please." He was sweating.

"Walter. you are just making it worse for yourself. If we're late for the restaurant because you refuse to accept your punishment then I shall be very angry indeed."

Clemmie (from *Clemmie* by John D. MacDonald)

Clemmie stretched and leaned back and smiled at him. "It's time I was married. Fitz. And you'll do nicely. You can have a lovely time being Clemmie's husband. But you won't own me. If I want to go out. I'll go out. And if I want to go on a trip. I'll go on a trip alone. You'll have no complaint coming. and no complaint to make. And you're going to try in every way you can to keep me from being bored. because you're going to learn that when I'm bored. I'm not pleasant to you. That will be a very simple conditioned reflex for you to acquire. And we will live precisely the way I want us to live. and there will never be any complaints. because you never had it so good. And if from time to time. you happen to feel any cute little horns sprouting. it's because you've been boring and stuffy and tiresome. As you have the last few days."

"Are you trying to admit what you did this afternoon?"

She got up quickly and walked over to him and stood

with her hands on her hips, her face tilted up. "Now, you see, you've made me angry, dear, and that's another thing. That's a thing to be especially avoided. You'll have to learn that..."

In keeping with 1950s American mores, MacDonald has this male character finally break free from Clemmie's clutches (after she tosses him a soiled pair of her nylons and lectures him in the finer points of hand-washing) and reassert his manhood, albeit shakily.

Eosuchus has no such qualms about female supremacy. Josie Brooks utterly triumphs over poor, broken Walter, as is made clear in the last seven words of the story: "...he bent before her in complete submission."

Both highly recommended.

Comments:

Enoch: MacDonald also wrote *The Girl, The Gold Watch and Everything* which had a character kinda similar to Clemmie who just overwhelmed and dominated the hapless protagonist for a short time. Of course, as with *Clemmie*, he "escapes" in the end.

Mark: Enoch, I'm impressed. I forgot that character. I'll have to reread it. It's one of my favorite sci-fi or speculative fiction stories. I just checked with IMDB and found the TV movie starring Robert Hays and Paw Dawber.

Enoch: The dominating woman's name was Charla, and she was after whatever his uncle's secret was (the gold watch, but she didn't know that).

Burnsie: I read "Have You Been a Good Boy?" by eosuchus intently. My wife asks me that very same question often. Now I want her to get home from work so bad because I have an overwhelming hunger to serve and please.

Woman on Top (7.25.08)

Women have been getting the upper hand for years on Madison Avenue, or wherever new advertising campaigns are incubated.

It's just getting edgier and more blatant, is all.

In a recent Cadillac commercial, "Khakis," a leggy young female exec revels in intimidating her male subordinates. The "climax" comes when her mere presence beside one of these guys in the elevator causes his ballpoint pen to spurt its load into his shirt pocket. ("Khakis" was named by *Adweek* one of its Best Spots of the Year.)

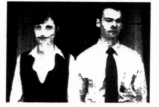

Nothing new here. "The Girl Wins" has been the rule in advertising for many years. Which means, of course, the Guy Loses. Other rules follow, as in Rock, Paper, Scissors, spelling out who trumps whom, in terms of gender, ethnicity, social status, in the careful hierarchy of political correctness.

Whether or not these rules of precedence are spelled out somewhere, they are definitely followed, tacitly and exactly.

It took Women's Lib to bring us *Thelma & Louise* and Sharon Stone uncrossing her legs to make her interrogators sweat in *Basic Instinct*. But demanding (and drop-dead gorgeous) women have had a long and profitable cinematic run... Theda Bara, Mae West, Joan Crawford, Bette Davis, Joan Collins come quickly to mind.

And what is more titillating to a male moviegoer (of any age) than watching some cinematic love goddess manifest her sexually aggressive side on the big screen? Like Marilyn Monroe not only seducing Tony Curtis in *Some Like It Hot*, but climbing all over him to do it? (Of course, he's an exceedingly willing "victim.")

Or the Great Greta Garbo looking lovingly down on John Gilbert, before wrapping an arm around his neck and pulling his willing mouth to hers?

Sometimes it's fun to be looking up... at the Goddess on Top.

May the trend continue.

POSTSCRIPT

Who Made YOU an Expert? (4.25.08)

Most of the comments I got from readers of the "Worshipping Your Wife" website, I'm happy to report, are truly appreciative. Which is why I went ahead and finished the darned book.

But, in the world's largest idea mall, you can't please everybody. So, every now and again I get contentious emails. Asking, like, Who made *you* an expert? What are your credentials? Do you have a degree in psych, behavioral science, sociology, anthropology? In anything?

C'mon. Do we really want to live in a regimented, regulated world where only approved and sanctioned "experts" are allowed to have an opinion, only highly credentialed pundits can pontificate? No, we don't. At least I don't. That's what's so refreshing and liberating about the Web. It lets me, like so many other unqualified, unwashed folk, speak my piece and call 'em as I see 'em in the free marketplace of ideas.

I'm reminded of the Jma 'el Fna, this huge square of beaten earth in the center of Marrakesh. It's a meeting of ancient caravan routes, a legendary Arab-Berber swapmeet, little changed over the centuries. You can still wander the stalls, feasting on roasted mutton, and find snake charmers and guys who'll yank a bad tooth with pliers or write you a love letter, side by side with sellers of pirated designer jeans, DVDs and junk jewelry. You pays your money and takes your choice. The Internet is like that.

POSTSCRIPT: WHO MADE *YOU* AN EXPERT?

Or there's the Speakers' Corner in London's Hyde Park. where the would-be orators line up every few feet. sounding off on every topic under the sun (as long as they're not too inciteful). Kind of like the blogosphere. which allows anyone with a cyber-soapbox to speak his or her mind. Wanderers-by can linger and listen. or just move on.

Who made me an expert on men and women. on marriage. or wife worship? Nobody. I'm just a guy who found something that worked miracles in his own marriage. then discovered from some other guys the same formula had worked miracles in their marriages.

So now I'm shouting the good news from the housetops. And I'm not gonna stop.

Comments:

Art: I've been voraciously reading every post starting with your most recent. I hereby commit to courtly behavior and am confident not only will it be its own reward but that my marriage will return to the heady days when we couldn't keep our hands off each other some 18 years ago. Thanks. Dr. Mark.

Mark: Art. can I quote your endorsement to my wife? Seriously. it means a lot to hear that some of my sincere scribblings are being enthusiastically received. and may even make a difference in terms of a husband's daily devotion to his wife. Good luck in your noble endeavor.

Art: It would be my honor. For once I'm not afraid who knows I'm pussywhipped (at least as described by you).

For Further Reading:

A great many online resources were cited, quoted or paraphrased in the preceding pages. For sake of brevity, I am listing here only a few "primary sources," all of which make excellent points of departure for readers interested in exploring further the wonderful world of female-led relationships. Just plug the names below into your favorite search engine and off you go.

Books and Blogs:
Around Her Finger by Emily and Ken Addison
Worshipping Your Wife by Mark Remond

Websites:
Lady Misato's "Real Women Don't Do Housework"
Elise Sutton's "Guide to Loving Female Authority"
Barbara Abernathy's "Venus On Top Society"

Message Boards:
Lady Misato's "Wife Worship Group" (Facebook)
"She Makes the Rules"

Printed in Great Britain
by Amazon.co.uk, Ltd.,
Marston Gate.